THE LATEST IN PERITONEAL DIALYSIS

Edited by **Abelardo Aguilera Peralta**

The Latest in Peritoneal Dialysis

http://dx.doi.org/10.5772/45910
Edited by Abelardo Aguilera Peralta

Contributors

Joseph C.K. Leung, Loretta Y Y Chan, Sydney C. W. Tang, Kar Neng Lai, Betül Kalender, Necmi Eren, Zhen Su, Niko Braun, Joerg Latus, Christoph Ulmer, Martin Kimmel, Dominik Alscher, Abelardo Isaac Aguilera Peralta

Published by InTech

Janeza Trdine 9, 51000 Rijeka, Croatia

Copyright © 2013 InTech

Notice

Publishing Process Manager Ana Pantar
Technical Editor InTech DTP team
Cover InTech Design team

Additional hard copies can be obtained from orders@intechopen.com

The Latest in Peritoneal Dialysis, Edited by Abelardo Aguilera Peralta
p. cm.
ISBN 978-953-51-1164-1

For EU product safety concerns:
IN TECH d.o.o., Prolaz Marije Krucifikse Kozulić 3, 51000 Rijeka, Croatia,
info@intechopen.com or visit our website at intechopen.com.

Meet the editor

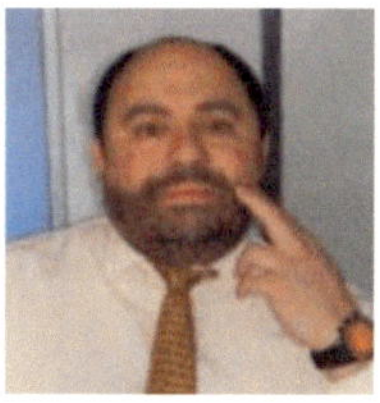

Dr. Abelardo Aguilera Peralta was born in Tegucigalpa, Honduras on June 3, 1967. He obtained the title of general practitioner in 1989 at the Facultad de Medicina de la Universidad Nacional Autónoma de Honduras, in Tegucigalpa. He studied Nephrology at the Hospital Ramón y Cajal, from Madrid, Spain (1991-1994) and obtained the title of Doctor (PhD) from the Universidad Autónoma de Madrid (2007). He was also a Pre-doctoral fellow at the Nephrology Institute, Cardiff, Wales, UK (1999-2000). Currently Dr. Aguilera is a senior researcher for the Miguel Servet Program at the Hospital Universitario de la Princesa, Madrid, since 2007. Dr. Aguilera has also more than 100 scientific articles published mainly in international journals, among which the New Engl J Med, J Am Soc Nephrol, Lab Investigation, Plos One, etc. He has received more than 25 national and international awards, has a degree in Physics. He is a specialist in family medicine and a Reviewer and editor of several international journals.
Finally, his main research areas are epithelial-to-mesenchymal transition of mesothelial cells and peritoneal membrane failure, and disorders in appetite regulation on dialysis patients.

Contents

Preface

The peritoneal dialysis (PD) is a kidney replacement therapy technique that has been growing in the last years. One reason for this growth is the freedom that the PD technique provides patients allowing them a better social development. However, parallel to the increase in frequency, it also increased its complications.

Cardiovascular and infectious diseases, malnutrition and peritoneal damage arising from inherent to PD process itself are still the leading causes of morbidity and mortality. Recently, there have been many advances in the understanding of the complications associated with PD and uremic state that suggests that the peritoneal cavity is a victim of the attacks produced by bioincompatible liquids, plastics, hemoperitoneum and infections and see victimizer because activation of this cavity acts as a true organ releasing substances with systemic effects. These substances could induce systemic effects as inflammation, dyslipidemia, diabetes, hypertension, accelerated atherosclerosis and malnutrition. Effectively, the hyperproduction and renal retention of pro-inflammatory cytokines is key for the initiation and maintenance of accelerated atherosclerosis, loss of renal function, bone renal diseases, protein malnutrition and other uremic complications. Furthermore, local effects of PD liquids that activate the immune system, the abdominal fat tissue, which is bathed by these PD liquids, the mesothelial cells and the other components of the abdominal cavity, induce deterioration of the peritoneal membrane reaching anatomical and functional failure. Although considerable efforts to improve the biocompatibility of PD fluid has been made in the last years. It should be noted also that the changes undergone in the peritoneal and mesothelial-to-mesenchymal transition (MMT) offer new and novel therapeutic opportunities. MMT is regularly triggered by the action of glucose degradation products, low pH of the PD fluids, and other advance glycation end-products formation. These transdifferentiated mesothelial cells acquire migratory capacity, invade the submesotelio where they produce high quantity of extracellular matrix components and high number of sanguineous and lymphatic vessels (angiogenesis and lymphangiogenesis).

This book provides an update on the emerging concepts in relation to new substances and mechanisms implicated in PD complications and attempts to organize the puzzle of these potentially active molecules. The authors have made a significant effort to update and summarize the relevance of each topic and especially to sort, in a logical and understandable way, the information provided here. New therapeutic strategies are proposed.

Dr. Abelardo Aguilera Peralta (MD, Ph.D),
specialty in Nephrology,
senior researcher (Miguel Servet Program)
at Instituto de Investigación Sanitaria del Hospital Universitaria de la Princesa,
Madrid, Spain

Section 1

The Peritoneal Catheter in Peritoneal Dialysis

Chapter 1

Peritoneal Dialysis Catheter Placement and Management

Zhen Su

Additional information is available at the end of the chapter

http://dx.doi.org/10.5772/56596

1. Introduction

Peritoneal dialysis (PD) is an alternative to hemodialysis in patients with end-stage renal disease (ESRD). The main function of a peritoneal dialysis catheter is to permit consistent bidirectional flow of dialysate into intraabdominal peritoneal cavity without obstruction or undue discomfort [1]. Most catheters are flexible tubes with multiple ports in the intraabdominal segment which is ideally positioned freely in the intraabdominal pelvic area. The catheter's function depends upon its design, implantation site, and the configuration of the system used to perform dialysis exchanges, and also be directly related to skill of catheter placement doctors, catheter-related problems and infections are responsible for approximately 20% of implantation technique failure [2]. 12 contents of this chapter are types of catheters, considerations in catheter placement, exit site location, exit site size, antibiotic prophylaxis, implantation technique, postoperative catheter care, exit site care, complication, repositioning migrated peritoneal dialysis catheters, brief information for patients, recommendations.

1.1. Types of catheters

Many types of catheters are currently available for chronic peritoneal dialysis (Figure 1).

Peritoneal catheters have intraperitoneal and extraperitoneal segments. The extraperitoneal segment passes through a tunnel within the abdominal wall, exits through the skin, and has an external segment. Most catheters are flexible tubes with multiple ports in the distal intraperitoneal segment. The intraperitoneal portion of the catheter should be ideally placed between the visceral and parietal peritoneum near the pouch of Douglas. The catheter's midportion is normally implanted within the wall of the abdomen by one to two Dacron velour cuffs. With double-cuffed catheters, the inner cuff should be imbedded in the abdominal rectus muscle to prevent leaks; the superficial cuff in both double cuff and single cuff catheters should

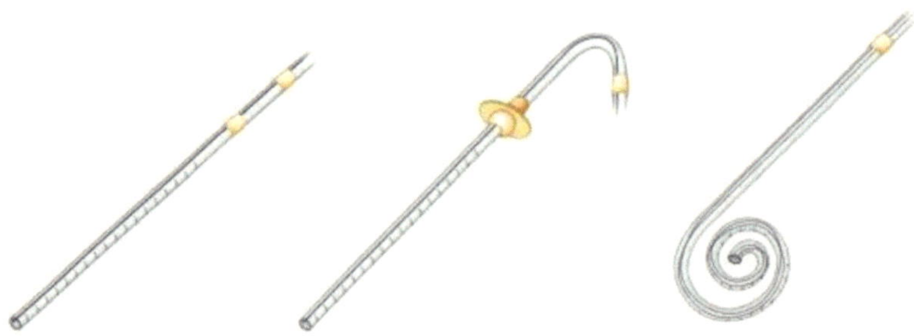

Figure 1. Intraperitoneal and extraperitoneal designs of currently available peritoneal catheters.

be placed subcutaneously approximately 2 cm from the catheter exit site on the abdominal wall to create a dead space in between the two cuffs, which is believed would prevent migration of infections coming from the exit site. Double cuff catheters have the advantages of fewer complications, a longer time to first peritonitis episode, and longer survival [3].More than 90% of the catheters used have two cuffs.

The double cuff straight Tenckhoff catheter, a silicone catheter with a straight intraabdominal portion is a most widely used catheter [4], followed by the swan-neck catheter [5]. The Tenckhoff and swan-neck catheters terminal segment is either straight or coiled. Catheters with a coiled intraperitoneal segment may minimize infusion and pressure pain. The straight double-cuff Tenckhoff catheter is about 40 cm long with an intraperitoneal segment about 15 cm long, an intramural segment about 5 to 7 cm long, and an external segment about 16 cm long. The open-ended intraperitoneal segment has multiple 0.5 mm side openings in the terminal 11 cm segment. Most Tenckhoff catheters have a barium-impregnated radiopaque stripe throughout the catheter length to assist in radiologic visualization. Overall catheter survival is approximately 88 percent at one year with removal rates of 15 percent per year [6].

The swan-neck catheter is a modified Tenckhoff catheter. The intraperitoneal segment of the swan-neck catheter is identical to that of the Tenckhoff catheter. The swan-neck catheter can be placed in a bend tunnel with both external and internal segments of the tunnel directed downwards. A long tunnel, downward-directed exit, and two intramural cuffs tend to reduce exit and tunnel infection rates. However, a study comparing swan-neck and straight Tenckhoff catheters have shown a similar risk for peritonitis and exit infection, but less cuff extrusion with the swan-neck design. The lower incidence of cuff extrusion enhances the survival of the swan-neck catheters [6]. The other catheters in use are the T-fluted catheter; the self-locating catheter; the Cruz catheter; the Toronto Western Hospital catheter; the Ash catheter; the column disc catheter; and the Gore-Tex peritoneal catheter [7].

Although all cause mortality may be lower with straight catheters, a review found no difference related to prevention of peritonitis with respect to straight versus coiled or single versus doubled cuffed catheters [8]. A randomized prospective study of 132 patients found no difference in dialysis adequacy measures between the coiled catheter group and straight catheter group [9]. A meta-analysis that compared swan neck catheters with a coiled versus a straight end showed no significant difference in overall catheter failure. However, late (>8 weeks) catheter tip migration was more common with the coiled end catheters [10].

Presternal catheters were designed to allow for an exit site in a presternal location. Patients with obesity, floppy abdominal skin folds, ostomies, or incontinence of urine or feces, children wearing diapers, are all indications to use an extended catheter system providing a remote exit site location to the upper abdomen or chest [11]. Exit site location of a presternal catheter should be at least 3 cm off the midline. A review showed a nonsignificant trend for improved survival and lower peritonitis rates was observed with presternal compared with abdominal catheters [12]. In a study of 200 patients, anthropometric analysis to help maximize the position of the catheter tip to a deep pelvic location and ideal exit site location found that the optimal catheter type may differ in men and women [13]. Swan neck catheters with a downwardly-directed external limb and exit site were better suited to females, while straight Tenckhoff catheters and a laterally-directed tunnel and exit site were better suited to males [14]. The gender differences primarily resulted from the location of the belt line combined with the desire to produce a downwardly-directed exit site. Thus, using a single, preferred catheter for all patients may not achieve ideal pelvic positioning of the catheter tip, it is not the optimal strategy.

Biofilm is an important factor in the development of PD catheter infections. It is no available catheter material resists biofilm formation now. Most available peritoneal catheters are made of either silicone rubber or polyurethane, there is little long-term experience with these catheters for PD.

Summary, it is no particular catheter is definitively better than the standard double cuff silicone Teckhoff catheter for the prevention of peritonitis [15].

2. Considerations in catheter placement

When inserting a peritoneal dialysis catheter, various factors (include the location of the exit site, use of prophylactic antibiotics, implantation technique, preoperative and postoperative care of the catheter, and temporal needs for dialysis [16]) require consideration.

3. Exit site location

The subcutaneous tract and exit site should face downward and laterally to avoid exit-site infection. Considering for patient comfort and accessibility to the catheter, therefore it is best to avoid exit sites over scars, belt lines, and skin folds. To determine the best location, it is often necessary to mark the desired location for the catheter's exit site with the patient in a sitting position and upright position, rather than when the patient is lying on the operation table awaiting catheter insertion. With the patient in the supine position, the position of the insertion site, is established by aligning the upper border of the symphysis pubis (a reliable landmark for the ideal position of the catheter tip in the true pelvis). Once the insertion site is determined, the appropriate catheter can be selected to produce a downwardly-directed tunnel and acceptable exit site location for the patient.

Most PD catheters are placed in a paramedian or lateral abdominal location rather than in the midline. A paramedian location also provides better structural support for and a strong seal around the catheter, thereby minimizing the risk of peritoneal leak. This location allows for positioning of the catheter's deep cuff in the rectus muscle, permitting better tissue ingrowth around the cuff due to the richer vascularization of muscle tissue.

We recommend that PD catheters be placed in a paramedian or lateral abdominal location rather than in the midline.

4. Exit site size

A prospective nonrandomized study found that the risks of first exit site and tunnel infections, catheter-related peritonitis, and catheter removal were associated with large exit site wounds [17]. Careful dissection and exit-site construction resulting in the smallest possible hole for the exiting catheter is therefore desirable.

Sutures should never be placed at the catheter exit site. Suture material may act as a nidus for bacterial growth and increase the risk of catheter-related infection. Fibroblast ingrowth of the Dacron cuff is sufficient to anchor the catheter, obviating the need for suture material at the exit site.

5. Antibiotic prophylaxis

A little data relating to the efficacy of an antibiotic just prior to peritoneal catheter placement may decrease the incidence of wound infection and peritonitis [18]. Four randomized prospective studies consisting of 335 patients found that the use of perioperative intravenous antibiotics, compared with no treatment, significantly reduced the risk of peritonitis within one month of surgery [19].

Vancomycin has a little renal toxicity, and a rise in the incidence of vancomycin resistant Enterococcus sp. Therefore, the routine use of vancomycin for prophylaxis prior to catheter insertion is not recommended. A first or second generation cephalosporin, such as a cephalosporin, should be the first choice [20].

We suggested that a single dose of a first or second generation cephalosporin should be given intravenously, vancomycin not to be routinely used.

6. Implantation technique

Compared with an upwardly or horizontally-directed PD catheter tunnel, a downwardly-directed tunnel is preferred and recommended by International Guidelines since it may be associated with fewer catheter infections and fewer peritonitis episodes resulting from catheter or tunnel infections [21]. Catheters with a permanent bend (eg, Swan Neck catheter) naturally have a downwardly-directed tunnel because of the catheter's configuration (Figure 1).

For long-term use, PD catheters such as the Tenckhoff or Swan-neck catheters can be inserted into the abdominal cavity by surgeons [22], experienced nephrologist [23]or interventional radiologists [24]. There are several techniques of PD catheter insertion: 1) surgical placement, either by a standard dissection or by a modification, such as the buried technique or using a presternally-located catheter; 2) laparoscopic [25], [26]; 3) fluoroscopic insertion [27], [28]; and 4) blind (Seldinger) [29], At the bedside, using a trocar and guidewire technique (generally reserved for temporary acute PD).

1. Surgery: Surgical placement of catheters has the advantage of precise catheter placement with little risk of viscus perforation. Disadvantages are the longer time involved (including operating room scheduling), greater cost, and larger incision required.

Technical Procedure:

Pre-operatively, the surgeon will have marked the exit place of the catheter together with the patient (left or right), well above the belt.

The patient will be operated under general anaesthesia or conscious sedation. Antibiotic prophylaxis will be administered on the ward approximately 1 hour before incision. Desinfection will routinely be applied. The patient will be covered with sterile drapes. The patient is put in Trendelenburg position. Insertion site will be selected to be 9~13 cm above the upper border of the symphysis pubis, and 2 cm to the left or right and lateral to the midline.

A 3~5cm skin incision is made, dissection is performed layer by layer to expose the anterior rectus sheath. The rectus muscle fibers are bluntly separated until the posterior sheath, and the peritoneum is then incised to create a small opening. The surgeon ensures that the surrounding peritoneum is free of adhesions. The catheter is introduced and the tip is placed in the pouch of Douglas. The internal cuff is secured within the rectus muscle, and then an absorbable purse-string suture completed the closure at the peritoneum and posterior rectus sheath. Testing of inflow and outflow is done. The proximal end of the catheter is connected to a tunneled needle, and a subcutaneous tunnel to the preferred exit site is created with tunneled needle. The tunneled needle is desirable to help prevent tunnel infection. The external cuff is placed subcutaneously at approximately 2 cm from the exit point. No sutures is placed at the skin exit. Free drainage of PD fluid is tested.

The buried catheter technique differs from the standard surgical technique, in that the extraperitoneal portion of the catheter is buried in the abdominal subcutaneous tissue until the patient is ready for PD, usually 4 to 6 weeks after catheter placement [30]. At that time, the catheter is exteriorized. This method was developed to possibly reduce peritonitis and catheter infections by allowing complete sinus tract healing and fibroblast ingrowth into the cuff. Most hospitals continue to use the standard technique unless early infection rates are high. The principal disadvantages of the buried technique are the need for two procedures and the longer waiting time for catheter use. Few randomized prospective trials have some conflicting results: In two prospective randomized study, the buried technique, compared with the standard technique, was not associated with a reduced risk of peritonitis or exit-site infection [31]; Another study of 214 new catheters (59 implanted using the buried technique and 155 via the conventional method) also showed no difference in peritonitis rates [32]. A third study of 349 buried catheters found that prolonged catheter embedding (131 to 2041 days) prior to exteriorization and use may lower the risk of initial infection of the tract [33].

The peritoneal catheter implantation technique is the same as the surgical insertion, except that the PD catheter has a straight design instead of a swan neck. After the PD catheter is placed, then a second catheter is tunneled from the mid-abdomen up to the chest wall. The two catheters are connected by a titanium joint piece. The second catheter has two cuffs. The exit site is located lateral to the mid-sternal line.

2. laparoscopy: Peritoneoscopic catheter placement permits to use immediately. For an experienced doctor, it is a relatively simple and quick procedure. At one center, a significantly lower incidence of flow dysfunction was observed with such placement (particularly advanced laparoscopic techniques) compared with an open surgical procedure [34].

Technical Procedure:

Peritoneal catheters placed peritoneoscopically are implanted through the rectus muscle using the Y-TEC peritoneoscope system. Under local anesthesia, a 2 cm skin incision is made. The subcutaneous tissue is dissected up to the rectus muscle. A catheter guide is inserted into the abdomen, and the Y-TEC peritoneoscope is inserted into the catheter to assess initial entry to the peritoneal cavity. The scope is removed, and 500 mL of air is infused into the cavity. The scope is again replaced and advanced to the pelvic area. This area is inspected for adhesions and bowel loops. The scope is again removed, and the peritoneal catheter is introduced through the catheter with the help of a stainless steel stylet. The catheter is advanced to the pelvic area. The stylet is removed, and the inner cuff is buried into the musculature. The exit location is determined, and the catheter is tunneled to that location.

3. Fluoroscopy: Percutaneous fluoroscopy-guided placement provides accurate placement with little waiting time and a relatively small incision [35], but the incidence of late leakage appears to be increased.

Technical Procedure:

An ultrasound machine with a 5~12MHz transducer and a sterile cover is used to guide a 21 gauge needle into the peritoneum. Under ultrasound guidance the needle penetrates through the skin, the subcutaneous tissue, the outer fascia of rectus muscle, the muscle fibers, the inner fascia, and the parietal layer of peritoneum. 3~5 mL contrast is injected into the peritoneal cavity under fluoroscopy to assure appropriate location. A radiologic pattern of outer bowel delineation is indicative of a good placement. A wire is introduced through the needle. The needle is exchanged for a 6 French catheter sheath. A 2 cm incision is made on the skin, and the subcutaneous tissue is digitally dissected up to the rectus muscle. A series of dilators are passed over a stiff glide wire, and an 18-French, peel-away sheath is placed. A peritoneal dialysis catheter is introduced over the stiff glide wire into the peritoneal cavity. The inner cuff is pushed into the muscle before removing the peel-away sheath. Alternatively, the tunnel could be created before catheter insertion into the peritoneum. A tunnel is created with an exit site located lateral, and below the initial incision with the outer cuff buried in the subcutaneous tissue. A final fluoroscopic imaging is performed to verify placement of the peritoneal catheter. Inflow and outflow of the PD catheter is tested with 500 mL of normal saline.

4. Bedside catheter placement: The benefits of bedside catheter placement technique require a small incision, quick and inexpensive, and permits immediate use. The shortcomings of primarily technical is a blind procedure, thereby resulting in a greater risk of inadvertent organ and vessel perforation; leaks and poor catheter flow are also common.

The type of catheter placement generally outweigh the advantages in most patients; exceptions include some cases of acute renal failure, and some individuals unable to tolerate the anesthesia required for catheter placement in the operating room. This method is not used for chronic catheter placement.

Summary, as with the choice of catheter, the technique used by a PD program depends upon the preferences and expertise of the surgeon or nephrologist inserting the catheter. Each method of insertion has its benefits, but no technique has been shown to be preferable overall [36]. Individual experience will dictate the technique and operators placing PD catheters.

7. Postoperative catheter care

Postoperative catheter care is very important. Patients stayed supine for the first 24 hours after catheter insertion. Usually PD is started between 2 and 3 weeks after placement of the catheter, to allow for wound healing, and securing of the catheter cuff. Providing sufficient time for healing, helps to avoid leaks, which can increase the risk of infection. Newly placed catheters are usually flushed with Low-volume dialysate until the effluent is clear. Then the catheter is capped and a dressing applied. If fibrin or clots are evident in effluent dialysate, heparin may be added as 500 to 1000 units/L dialysate. As the heparin is not peritoneally absorbed, some may choose to "lock" the PD catheter with heparin during temporary cessation of PD in an attempt to avoid clotting of the PD catheter. Others may elect not to lock the PD catheter as the risk of catheter occlusion during non-use is probably low.

A 1000mL volume of dialysis solution is used for supine PD exchanges if immediate dialysis is needed. If PD is required less than 10 days following catheter placement, less than 1500 mL volume exchanges performed in the recumbent position only can be performed with little risk of a significant leak. However, a single center study showed that the catheter may be used immediately after placement without increasing the risk of infection, the leaks were minor, urgent initiation was associated with no greater risk of peritonitis or exit site infection at three months [37].

These optimal catheter care post-placement are that the catheter site be covered with nonocclusive dressing and remain undisturbed for 10 to 14 days. The catheter should be immobilized with a dressing. Infrequent dressing changes (such as once/week) are probably sufficient for the first one to two weeks after implantation.

8. Exit site care

Optimal care and cleaning of the exit site is unknown. There are few prospective, controlled trials comparing agents to clean PD catheter exit sites.

9. Complication

A major complication during placement of the PD catheter is bowel perforation. It is infrequent with all techniques except for blind placement, but once identified, it requires bowel rest, intravenous antibiotic therapy, and rarely surgical exploration [38]. PD leaks around the catheter less than 10% [39]. Prophylactic antibiotics are usually given, perioperative infection and bleeding are rare. Tip migration is a very common (up to 35%) late complication, which could cause problems with draining of the PD fluid. It can be fixed with either radiologic or surgical manipulation [40], or non-traumatic maneuver [41].

Multiple abdominal surgeries may be complicated by the presence of dense intra-abdominal adhesions, due in part to repeated peritonitis episodes. Hemodialysis may be required in the immediate post-operative period depending upon the patient's clinical status, degree of residual renal function, and ability to perform supine only, low volume PD exchanges. Resumption of peritoneal dialysis after a week delay is reasonable.

As with all patients, patients with autosomal dominant polycystic kidney disease (ADPKD) who progress to ESRD require either dialysis or renal transplantation. Because massively enlarged kidneys make it difficult for the ADPKD patients to accommodate large volumes of peritoneal dialysate fluid. In addition, there may be an increased risk of peritonitis secondary to cyst infections [42], patients with ADPKD and renal failure are therefore most commonly treated with hemodialysis or undergo renal transplantation, peritoneal dialysis is less commonly performed. However, a survival benefit among patients with ADPKD, compared to those without ADPKD, was observed with peritoneal dialysis; Limited evidence suggests that patients with ADPKD may have superior survival rates with peritoneal dialysis than with hemodialysis [43]. Some centers have also found that peritoneal dialysis is well tolerated and results in no specific difficulties in the patient with ADPKD who have reached ESRD [44].

10. Repositioning migrated peritoneal dialysis catheters

PD catheter migration refers to displacement of the PD catheter from the pelvis to the upper abdomen, often resulting in PD failure and catheter removal. The most common management technique for the migrated PD catheter at present is repositioning the catheter by laparoscopy [45], or surgically, which often causes more suffering and economic burden to the patient. We found an original non-traumatic maneuver for repositioning a migrated peritoneal dialysis catheter. Laxatives have a possible effect on the mobilization of misplaced catheters prior to maneuver.

Technical Procedure:

Our method includes dissociation, determination of the return route, and manual repositioning.

Dissociation: After the migration position is confirmed by abdominal x-ray, some of the dialysate is drained, with about 1000 mL retained in the abdomen. The patient lies, flexing the knees and relaxing the abdominal muscle. The operator stands on the right side of the patient, with the right hand feeling the site of the migrated catheter, which will cause a painful sensation in most patients. Feeling should be from a light force to a heavy force, and from the center to the periphery in clockwise and anticlockwise directions alternately for 20 times until the pain at the site of migration is significantly lessened. Again, using the pain point as the center, one hand presses the catheter and the other hand gives a gentle force in an upward radiating and right-to-left direction to dissociate the greater omentum, which might be wrapped around the catheter.

Determination of the Return Route: A return route is designed according the position of the catheter on the x-ray films. For patients with catheter migration to the right or left upper quadrant or the right lumbar region, the catheter is first moved toward the epigastrium and then repositioned downward. For patients with catheter migration to the epigastrium, repositioning is done directly downward. For patients with catheter migration to the left lumbar region, repositioning is done according to the size of the abdominal cavity: for patients with a big abdominal cavity, repositioning is implemented by pushing the catheter down to the left lower quadrant and then to the pelvic fossa; for patients with a small abdominal cavity, the catheter is first moved to the epigastrium and then downward to the pelvic fossa. For patients with catheter migration to the right or left iliac fossa, repositioning is implemented by moving the catheter directly to the pelvic fossa.

Manual Repositioning (Figure 2): For catheter migration to the right or left upper quadrant or the right lumbar region, the patient is asked to lie in a side position opposite to the migration, that is, a left-side position for right migration and vice versa.

Step 1: Pressing: The patient lies flat and the operator stands on the side of migration and uses both of his/her thumbs or the heel of the hand to press the intestine below the catheter tip, gently but vigorously shaking up and churning the abdominal contents, and using some directional pressure to facilitate gravity and the natural resiliency forces of the displaced

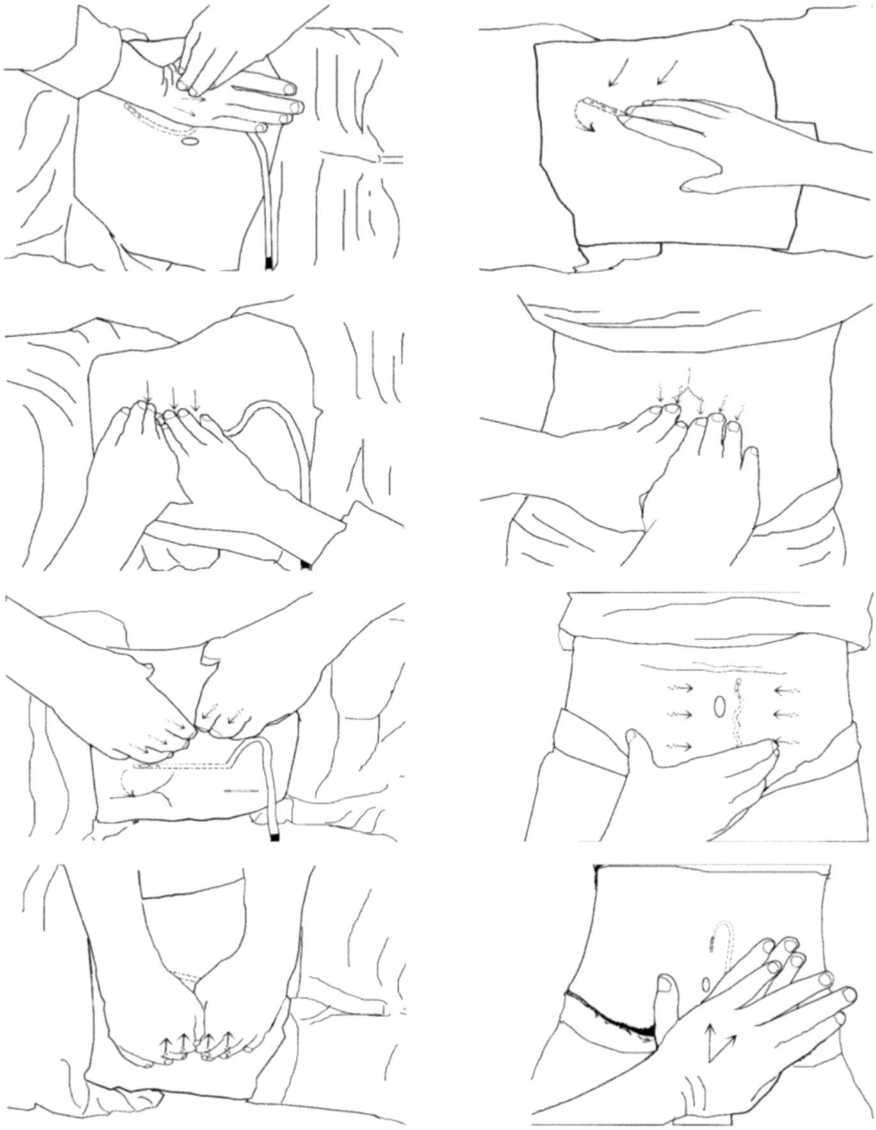

Figure 2. Steps in manual repositioning of a migrated peritoneal dialysis catheter.

catheter tubing to return it to the original pelvic position. This method is especially important for patients using coiled PD catheters.

Step 2: Palpating: The patient lies flat and the operator stands on the side opposite the migration, puts the left hand on the right hand, uses finger tips of both hands to feel and palpate the catheter with fluctuation of the patient's deep breathing, and at the same time pushes the catheter to the mid-axial line for 20 times.

Step 3: Vibrating: The operator stands behind the patient with the fingertips of both hands flexing naturally, vibrating the patient's abdominal wall at the site above the catheter at a rate of 180~200 times/minute, to a depth of 4~5 cm, for 3 minutes continuously.

Step 4: Wave Vibrating: The patient lies on his side and the operator stands behind the patient with the fingers of both hands holding the contralateral abdominal wall, vibrating the abdominal wall upwardly at a rate of 150 times/minute for 3 minutes.

Step 5: Rotating: The patient lies on his side and the operator extends the fingers of both hands widely, grasps both sides of the rectus abdominis, and rotates the abdominal wall in the direction opposite to migration at a rate of 100 times/minute for 2 minutes for the purpose of helping the intestine and the dialysate in the abdominal cavity move in a direction opposite to catheter migration and causing the catheter to move to the mid-axial line.

When the catheter is moved to the epigastrium through the above five steps, the patient is allowed to sit up and lean slightly backward, with the upper limbs resting on the arms of the chair, both knees flexing, the feet touching the ground, and the whole body relaxing naturally.

Step 6: Back-Pushing and Vibrating: The operator squats, with both hands moving forcefully downward as in Step 3.

Step 7: Swaying: The operator extends the fingers of both hands widely, grasps both sides of the rectus abdominis, and sways the abdominal wall left and right at a rate of 150 times/minute for 2 minutes.

Step 8: Compressing: The operator squats, overlaps both hands, places the heel of the hand on the anterior pubic symphysis, and then compresses the abdominal cavity in a superior–posterior direction at a rate of 100 times/minute for 2 minutes.

The above 8 steps are a set of actions and should be done completely for each repositioning, which lasts about 20 minutes. It is preferable to select the time point before replacing the dialysate for the sake of saving the dialysate.

For patients with catheter migration to the right or left iliac fossa or to the left lumbar region, and with a big abdominal cavity, steps 1, 2, 3, 5, 6, and 7 are enough, using the same frequency and duration as mentioned above. For patients with catheter migration to the epigastrium, steps 6~8 are sufficient but the duration should be doubled.

After completion of manual repositioning, the remaining 1000 mL dialysate is drained and replaced with fresh dialysate. During infusion of the dialysate, it is better to ask the patient to stand up and sit down 30~50 times, with both hands supporting the waist to facilitate catheter repositioning.

If the procedure has been successful and the amount and rate of dialysate flow has returned to the level before migration, the patient may have a sensation of perianal pressure by the end of drainage, which can be used as a clinical criterion for successful repositioning. If repositioning is successful on the first attempt, radiological examination is done the following day to confirm. If repositioning cannot be achieved on the first attempt, it can be repeated two to three times on the same day; and if repositioning cannot be achieved within a day, the procedure can be repeated on 3 consecutive days.

The present method is suitable for patients of all ages and body shapes, as long as their condition is stable. It is a safe, effective, economical, and painless maneuver to reposition the migrated PD catheter as an alternative to surgical intervention. We suggest that, once the diagnosis of catheter migration is confirmed, it is preferable to reposition the migrated catheter manually before endoscopic or surgical intervention

11. Brief information for patients

1. The catheter is placed on the left of the umbilicus. The patient may be given general or local anesthesia before the insertion procedure.

2. Although the catheter can be used right away, it is best to wait 10 to 14 days after placement before dialysis is performed, this method allows the catheter site to heal. In some hospital, a small volume of fluid can be exchanged during this time.

3. Care of the catheter and the skin around the catheter is important to keep the catheter functioning and also to minimize the risk of developing an infection. After the catheter is inserted, the insertion site is usually covered with a gauze dressing and tape to prevent the catheter from moving and keep the area clean. The dressing is usually changed at 7 to 10 days after placement. If a dressing change is needed before this time, it should be done using sterile techniques. The catheter should not be moved or handled excessively because this can increase the risk of infection. The area should be kept dry until it is well healed, usually for 10 to 14 days. This means that you should not take a shower or bath or go swimming during this time. You will be asked to limit lifting and vigorous exercise within three weeks.

4. Avoid constipation Straining to move the bowels can increase the risk of developing a hernia. Constipation, not moving the bowels regularly, can lead to catheter function problems (such as slow drain time, difficulty draining). To avoid constipation, your need a High-fiber diet, as well as a stool softener or laxative.

12. Recommendations

1. Many types of catheters are available for chronic peritoneal dialysis. The catheter used by a PD program primarily depends upon the preferences and experience of the clinician inserting the catheters, with some guidelines stating that no particular catheter is definitively better. However, we prefer double cuff catheters over single cuff catheters since double cuff catheters have the advantages of fewer complications, a longer time to first peritonitis episode, and longer survival.

2. As with the choice of catheter, the technique used by a PD program depends upon the preferences and expertise of the surgeon or nephrologist inserting the catheter. Each method of insertion has its benefits and shortage, but no technique has been shown to be preferable overall.

3. We recommend that PD catheters be placed in a paramedian or lateral abdominal location rather than in the midline. A downwardly-directed tunnel is preferred and prophylactic antibiotics should be given at the time of catheter placement.

Author details

Zhen Su*

Division of Nephrology, The First Affiliated Hospital of Wenzhou Medical University, Wenzhou, Zhejiang, China

References

[1] Cruz, C. The peritoneal dialysis catheter. Semin Dial 1995; 8:103.

[2] Flanigan M, Gokal R. Peritoneal catheters and exit-site practices toward optimum peritoneal access: A review of current developments. Perit Dial Int 2005; 25:132-139.

[3] Warady BA, Sullivan EK, Alexander SR. Lessons from the peritoneal dialysis patient database: a report of the North American Pediatric Renal Transplant Cooperative Study. Kidney Int Suppl 1996; 53:S68.

[4] Gokal R, Alexander S, Ash S, et al. Peritoneal catheters and exit-site practices toward optimum peritoneal access: 1998 update. Perit Dial Int 1998; 18:11.

[5] Negoi D, Prowant B.F, Twardowski Z.J. Current trends in the use of peritoneal dialysis catheters. Adv Perit Dial 2006; 22:147-152.

[6] Eklund B.H, Honkanen E.O, Kala A.R, et al. Peritoneal dialysis access: prospective randomized comparison of the swan neck and Tenckhoff catheters. Perit Dial Int 1995; 15:353-356.

[7] Kathuria P, Twardowski Z.J, Nichols W.K. Peritoneal dialysis access and exit-site care including surgical aspects. In: Khanna R, Krediet R, ed. Nolph and Gokal's textbook of peritoneal dialysis, 3rd ed. New York: Springer; 2009:371-446.

[8] Strippoli GF, Tong A, Johnson D, et al. Catheter-related interventions to prevent peritonitis in peritoneal dialysis: a systematic review of randomized, controlled trials. J Am Soc Nephrol 2004; 15:2735.

[9] Johnson DW, Wong J, Wiggins KJ, et al. A randomized controlled trial of coiled versus straight swan-neck Tenckh off catheters in peritoneal dialysis patients. Am J Kidney Dis 2006; 48:812.

[10] Xie J, Kiryluk K, Ren H, et al. Coiled versus straight peritoneal dialysis catheters: a randomized controlled trial and meta-analysis. Am J Kidney Dis 2011; 58:946.

[11] Twardowski Z.J. Presternal peritoneal catheter. Adv Ren Replace Ther 2002; 9:125-132.

[12] Twardowski ZJ, Prowant BF, Nichols WK, et al. Six-year experience with Swan neck presternal peritoneal dialysis catheter. Perit Dial Int 1998; 18:598.

[13] Crabtree JH, Burchette RJ, Siddiqi NA. Optimal peritoneal dialysis catheter type and exit site location: an anthropometric analysis. ASAIO J 2005; 51:743.

[14] Crabtree, JH. Selected best demonstrated practices in peritoneal dialysis access. Kidney Int 2006; 70:S27.

[15] Piraino B, Bailie GR, Bernardini J, et al. Peritoneal dialysis-related infections recommendations: 2005 update. Perit Dial Int 2005; 25:107.

[16] Ash SR. Chronic peritoneal dialysis catheters: overview of design, placement, and removal procedures. Semin Dial 2003; 16:323.

[17] Crabtree JH, Fishman A, Siddiqi RA, et al. The risk of infection and peritoneal catheter loss from implant procedure exit-site trauma. Perit Dial Int 1999; 19:366.

[18] European Best Practice Guidelines for peritoneal dialysis. Nephrol Dial Transplant 2005; 20(Suppl 9):3.

[19] Strippoli GF, Tong A, Johnson D, et al. Antimicrobial agents to prevent peritonitis in peritoneal dialysis: a systematic review of randomized controlled trials. Am J Kidney Dis 2004; 44:591.

[20] Keane WF, Bailie GR, Boeschoten E, et al. Adult peritoneal dialysis-related peritonitis treatment recommendations: 2000 update. Perit Dial Int 2000; 20:396.

[21] Flanigan M, Gokal R. Peritoneal catheters and exit-site practices toward optimum peritoneal access: a review of current developments. Perit Dial Int 2005; 25:132.

[22] Soontrapornchai P, Simapatanapong T. Comparison of open and laparoscopic secure placement of peritoneal dialysis catheters. Surg Endosc 2005; 19:137-139.

[23] Zaman F, Pervez A, Atray N.K, et al. Fluoroscopy-associated placement of peritoneal dialysis catheters by nephrologists. Semin Dial 2005; 18:247-251.

[24] Degesys G.E, Miller G.A, Ford K.K, et al. Tenckhoff peritoneal dialysis catheters: the use of fluoroscopy in management. Radiology 1985; 154:819-820.

[25] Tsimoyiannis E.C, Siakas P, Glantzounis G, et al. Laparoscopic placement of the Tenckhoff catheter for peritoneal dialysis. Surg Laparosc Endosc Percutan Tech 2000; 10:218-221.

[26] Crabtree JH, Fishman A. A laparoscopic method for optimal peritoneal dialysis access. Am Surg 2005; 71:135.

[27] Zaman F, Pervez A, Atray N.K, et al. Fluoroscopy-associated placement of peritoneal dialysis catheters by nephrologists. Semin Dial 2005; 18:247-251.

[28] Moon JY, Song S, Jung KH, et al. Fluoroscopically guided peritoneal dialysis catheter placement: long-term results from a single center. Perit Dial Int 2008; 28:163.

[29] Zappacosta A.R, Perras S.T, Closkey G.M. Seldinger technique for Tenckhoff catheter placement. ASAIO Trans 1991; 37:13-15.

[30] Moncrief JW, Popovich RP, Seare W, et al. Peritoneal dialysis access technology: the Austin Diagnostic Clinic experience. Perit Dial Int 1996; 16 Suppl 1:S327.

[31] Danielsson A, Blohmé L, Tranaeus A, et al. A prospective randomized study of the effect of a subcutaneously "buried" peritoneal dialysis catheter technique versus standard technique on the incidence of peritonitis and exit-site infection. Perit Dial Int 2002; 22:211.

[32] Wu CC, Su PF, Chiang SS. A prospective study to compare subcutaneously buried peritoneal dialysis catheter technique with conventional technique. Blood Purif 2007; 25:229.

[33] Brown PA, McCormick BB, Knoll G, et al. Complications and catheter survival with prolonged embedding of peritoneal dialysis catheters. Nephrol Dial Transplant 2008; 23:2299.

[34] Wright MJ, Bel'eed K, Johnson BF, et al. Randomized prospective comparison of laparoscopic and open peritoneal dialysis catheter insertion. Perit Dial Int 1999; 19:372.

[35] Moon JY, Song S, Jung KH, et al. Fluoroscopically guided peritoneal dialysis catheter placement: long-term results from a single center. Perit Dial Int 2008; 28:163.

[36] Strippoli GF, Tong A, Johnson D, et al. Catheter-related interventions to prevent peritonitis in peritoneal dialysis: a systematic review of randomized, controlled trials. J Am Soc Nephrol 2004; 15:2735.

[37] Ghaffari A. Urgent-start peritoneal dialysis: a quality improvement report. Am J Kidney Dis 2012; 59:400.

[38] Asif A, Byers P, Vieira C.E, et al. Peritoneoscopic placement of peritoneal dialysis catheter and bowel perforation: experience of an interventional nephrology program. Am J Kidney Dis 2003; 42:1270-1274.

[39] Ash S.R. Chronic peritoneal dialysis catheters: overview of design, placement, and review procedures. Semin Dial 2003; 16:323-334.

[40] Gadallah M.F, Arora N, Arumugam R, et al. Role of Fogarty catheter manipulation in management of migrate, nonfunctional peritoneal dialysis catheters. Am J Kidney Dis 2000; 35:301-305.

[41] Tu WT, Su Z, Shan YS. An original non-traumatic maneuver for repositioning migrated peritoneal dialysis catheters. Perit Dial Int. 2009;29:325-329.

[42] Lederman ED, McCoy G, Conti DJ, et al. Diverticulitis and polycystic kidney disease. Am Surg 2000; 66:200.

[43] Abbott KC, Agodoa LY. Polycystic kidney disease at end-stage renal disease in the United States: patient characteristics and survival. Clin Nephrol 2002; 57:208.

[44] Hadimeri H, Johansson AC, Haraldsson B, Nyberg G. CAPD in patients with autosomal dominant polycystic kidney disease. Perit Dial Int 1998; 18:429.

[45] Yilmazlar T, Kirdak T, Bilgin S, et al. Laparoscopic findings of peritoneal dialysis catheter malfunction and management outcomes. Perit Dial Int 2006;26: 374-379.

Section 2

Peritoneal Membrane Complication in Peritoneal Dialysis

Chapter 2

The Mesothelial to Mesenchymal Transition a Pathogenic and Therapeutic Key for Peritoneal Membrane Failure

Abelardo Aguilera, Jesús Loureiro,
Guadalupe Gónzalez-Mateo, Rafael Selgas and
Manuel López-Cabrera

Additional information is available at the end of the chapter

http://dx.doi.org/10.5772/56598

1. Introduction

Peritoneal dialysis (PD) is a form of renal replacement therapy that is growing progressively, possibly because of the freedom it offers to the patients and the undoubted improvement in the PD technique. Parallel the PD-related complications have also increased. In PD, the peritoneal membrane (PM) is exposed to bio-incompatible dialysis solutions, rich in glucose, which can cause peritoneal injury when associated with peritoneal incidents like repeated episodes of peritonitis or hemoperitoneum [1]. Progressive fibrosis, angiogenesis and ultimately, ultrafiltration failure, are some characteristics of the so-called sclerotic peritonitis syndromes (SPS) [2].

Several pathologic factors, such as inflammatory mediators, high glucose content, the presence of glucose degradation products, and low pH can induce peritoneal mesothelial cells (MCs) to lose certain epithelial characteristics, and they progressively acquire a fibroblast-like phenotype soon after initiation of PD [3]. This so-called mesothelial-to-mesenchymal transition (MMT) serves as a trigger for peritoneal fibrosis and angiogenesis, via up-regulation of transforming growth factor-β (TGF-β1 and vascular endothelial growth factor (VEGF), respectively. As such, MMT is considered an important potential therapeutic target in sclerotic peritonitis syndromes [4]. Encapsulating peritoneal sclerosis (EPS) is a severe form of peritoneal fibrosis characterized by intestinal encapsulation through the formation of excessive matrix components that subsequently may lead to obstruction of the intestinal tract [5]. Although rare, EPS is a serious complication of PD for which no specific and definitive treatment exists [6]. However, peritoneal resting, steroids, immunosuppressive agents and Tamoxifen have been used previously as therapeutic approaches with divergent results [4]. Herein, we review in detail the effect of PD liquids and other peritoneal accidents like peritonitis and hemoperitoneum on the MCs physiology, the trandifferentiation in fibroblast-like cells (MMT), its clinical correlation with data from peritoneal and morphologic function (peritoneal biopsies), the initiation and perpetuation of peritoneal fibrosis (SPS) and his eventual rise to EPS. We also purpose therapeutic alternatives, ranging from the improvement in the biocompatibility of the liquids of DP, the use of drugs available on the market today, or even the use of molecular strategies, as blockades or stimulation of genes involved in the peritoneal damage.

2. Morphologic and phenotypic MCs characterization

The mesothelium is a continuous superficial layer of MCs formed by flattened, polygonal, mononuclear, squamous epithelial cells. This monolayer shows remarkable fibrinolytic properties and is thought to be involved in the prevention of fibrous adhesion formation in the peritoneum. MCs cells have vast biosynthetic capacity and secrete phospholipids and phosphotidylcholine in the form of lamellar bodies that provide a lubricating surface for the movement of abdominal viscera [7]. Besides this function, the mesothelium also modulates peritoneal microcirculation by secreting vasodilators (eg, prostaglandin E2 and nitric oxide), as well as vasoconstrictors (eg, endothelin) [8]. The luminal aspect of MCs plasmalemma has numerous cytoplasmic extensions called "microvilli" which play a significant role in the transperitoneal transfer of anionic macromolecules such as proteins. Microvilli are extremely sensitive and easily lost due to injury [9].

MCs can be isolated from healthy omentum donors of elective abdominal surgeries and the effluent from patients with PD. The analysis of the effluent drained peritoneal MCs has allowed us to assess the health status of peritoneal. The purity of effluent and omentum-derived MC cultures are determined by the expression of standard mesothelial markers: ICAM-1, cytokeratins, and calretinine. MCs cultures remain stable, without any evident sign of senescence, for at least two to three passages [10, 11].

The analysis of cytokeratins and E-cadherin expression, that are typical epithelial markers and highly expressed in MC, is important to determine more precisely the nature of effluent-derived cells. High expression of cytokeratins and E-cadherin is only observed in omentum-derived MC, whereas effluent-derived cells show a progressive reduction in the expression of these molecules, although even fibroblast-like MC may maintain a small population of positive cells (Figure 1). In mixed populations the expression of cytokeratins and E-Cadherin is normally bimodal. Fibroblasts are completely negative for these two markers. Previous studies had characterized the cobblestone-like MC from effluents as indistinguishable from omentum-derived MC. However, already in this early stage a loss of apico-basolateral polarity as well as down-regulation of cytokeratins and E-Cadherin is observed *ex vivo*, even though cells still show a morphologically epithelioid appearance [10-12].

MCs Phenotype

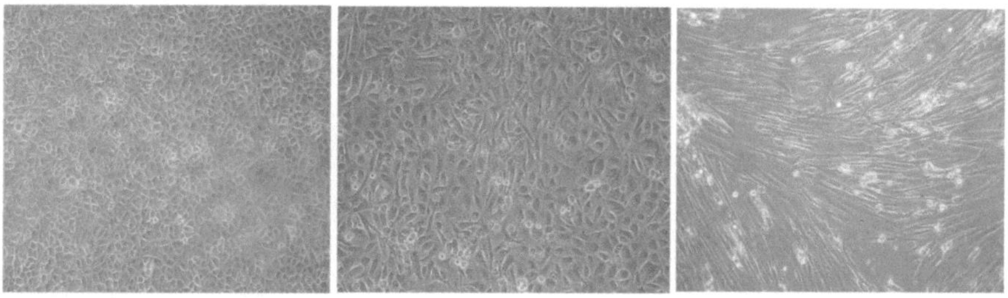

	Cobblestome (omentum)	Transitional (PD effluent)	Fibroblastic (PD effluent)
E-cadherin	+++	+	–
Snail (mRNA)	–	+/–	+++
ICAM-I	+++	+++	+++
Cytokeratins	+++	++	+/–
Calretinin	+++	++	+/–
Vimentin	+	++	+++
CA125	+++	+++	+++
VEGF	+	++	+++
Fibronectin	+/–	+	+++
Collagen I	+/–	+	+++
a-SMA	–	+/–	++
CTGF	+	+	?
TGF-b	+	+	?
N-cadherin	–	+	++
CD34	–	–	–

Figure 1. Morphology and gene expression of MCs. Panel "A" shows a culture of MCs isolated from omentum donor. Cells show the typical cobblestone phenotype. Panel "B" shows MCs isolated from PD effluent with transitional phenotype, and panel "C" shows a fibroblastoid phenotype these cells were isolated and cultured from the PD effluent. The genetic pattern of each phenotype is described below.

The morphological changes and down-regulation of cytokeratin and E-Cadherin in effluent-derived MC are indicative of an MMT. MMT is a complex and generally reversible process that starts with the disruption of intercellular junctions and loss of apical–basolateral polarity, typical of epithelial cells, which are then transformed into fibroblast-like cells with increased migratory, invasive and fibrogenic features. The objective of this process is to repair tissue wounds by promoting the recovery of ancestor capabilities of epithelial cells. Cell migration, production of extracellular matrix and induction of neoangiogenesis are the main activities [11, 12]. This process is conducted by the transforming growth factor-β (TGF-β) and the representative cell form is the myofibroblast (Figure 2). TGF-β synthesis may be stimulated by glucose, and infections, via peritoneal leucocyte-derived factors. TGF-β has been found to be up-regulated in peritoneal inflammatory processes and its over-expression has been correlated to worse PD outcomes [13]. Moreover, the injection of an adenovirus vector that transferred active TGF-β1 in rat and mice peritoneum induces myofibroblastic conversion of MC. [14, 15]. TGF-β is a growth factor that has been implicated as the causal agent in fibrosis of different tissues and organs [16].

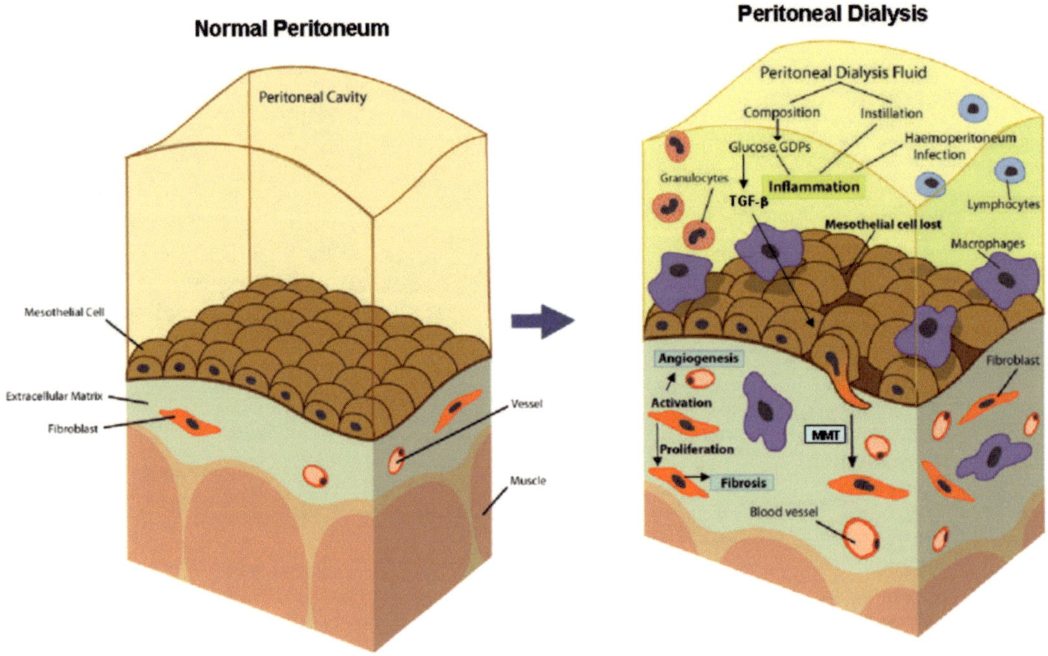

Figure 2. From a normal peritoneum to a PD peritoneum suffering MMT. Panel "A" shows a normal peritoneun without fibrosis, angiogenesis or MMT (3D image). Panel "B" shows a PD paritoneum with MCs exposed to PD fluids. MCs lose their microvilli, suffer MMT and invade submesothelial area, where synthesize VEGF, angiogenesis, proliferation, migration and EMC production. Both glucose (GDPs and AGEs) from PD fluids and inflammatory molecules stimulate TGF-β production which trigger MMT.

3. MMT signalling

Figure 3 shows the signaling cascade of MMT which begins with the activation of TGF-β which is considered the master molecule in peritoneal injury during PD. Activation of TGF-β receptors triggers smads-dependent and smads-independent signaling. Smads depending pathway include integrin-linked kinase, GSK-3, β-catenin, Lef-1/Tcf and AP gene cascade. Smads independing include RhoAp160ROCK and H-Ras/Raf/ ERK pathways [17-32].

4. Clinical implication of MMT in PM failure

We have described three major morphologies of MCs cultures from PD effluents: cobblestone-like, similar to omentum-derived MC, transitional and fibroblast-like MC which remained stable for at least two to three cell passages. After analyzing more than two hundred MC cultures with growth capacity, from more than 100 PD patients, we determined that the frequencies of the different effluent-derived MC cultures are approximately 53 percent for

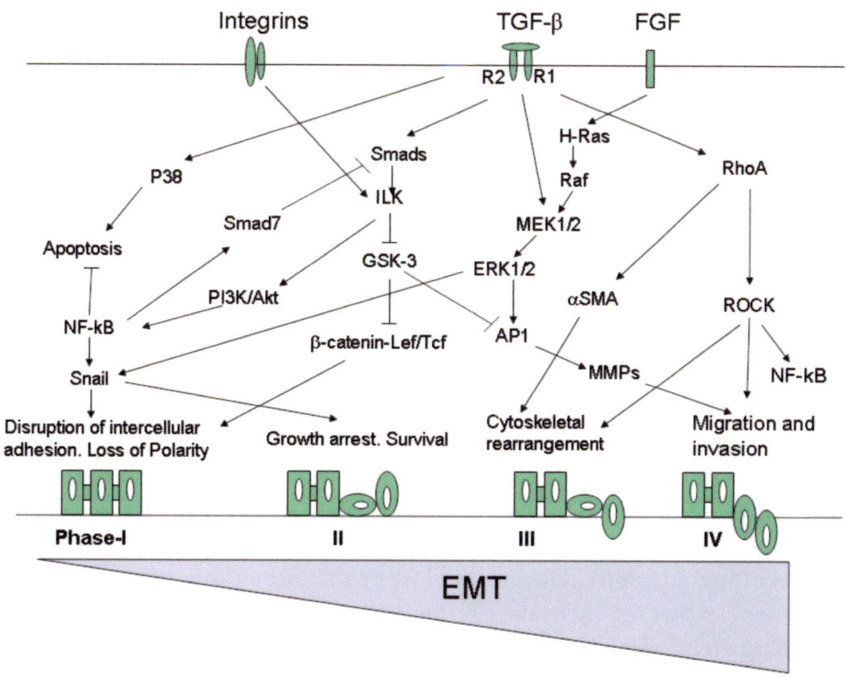

Figure 3. TGF-β signaling. Glucose, low pH from PD fluids, advanced glycation end products (AGEs), glucose degradation products (GDPs), peritonitis and haemoperitoneum stimulate TGF-β synthesis, and possibly FGF which in turn triggers the healing processes that ultimately lead to tissue fibrosis and angiogenesis. The increase in total VEGF production might increase the VEGF-C levels, which are directly implicated in lymphogenesis. TGF-β receptor I phosphorylates Smad 2 and 3 inducing their association with the common partner Smad 4, and then they translocate into the nucleus, where they control the expression of TGF-β-responsive genes, such as that encoding integrin-linked kinase (ILK). The activation of up-regulated ILK by β1 integrins results in strong phosphorylation of Akt and glycogen synthase kinase-3 (GSK-3). Phosphorylated-Akt triggers NF-kB activation, which in turn induces the expression of Smad 7, an inhibitory Smad molecule that interferes with the phosporylation of Smad 2 and 3, and of snail, a key regulator of MMT. The transcription factor snail regulates MMT by inhibiting the expression of E-cadherin, and by inducing growth arrest and survival, which confer selective advantage to migrating trans-differentiated cells. The phosphorylation of GSK-3 by ILK results in its inhibition and subsequent stabilization of β-catenin, released from the adherens junction, and of AP-1. Stabilized b-catenin, in conjunction with Lef-1/Tcf, may per se induce MMT, and AP-1 activates MMP-9 expression inducing the invasion of ECM. One of the main Smad-independent signalling cascades triggered by TGF-β receptor I ligation, includes the RhoAp160ROCK pathway that regulates cytoskeleton remodelling and cellular migration/ invasion. In addition, RhoA induces the expression of α-SMA in a ROCK-independent manner. Another signal transduction stimulated by TGF-β is the H-Ras/Raf/ ERK pathway, which is also necessary for the induction of snail expression and MMT.

cobblestone-like, 24 percent for transitional, and 17 percent for fibroblast-like MC. The prevalence of non-epitheliod MC cultures (transitional or fibroblast-like) is associated with the time the patients have been subjected to PD and with the episodes of acute or recurrent peritonitis or hemoperitoneum [3, 10, 11]. We have also described a less frequent (less than 6 percent) cell culture with mixed morphologies [3, 10]. Effluent mesothelial cells were isolated from 37 PD patients and analyzed for mesenchymal conversion. Mass transfer coefficient for creatinine (Cr-MTC) was used to evaluate peritoneal function. VEGF concentration was measured by using standard procedures. Patients whose drainage contained nonepithelioid mesothelial cells had greater serum VEGF levels than those with epithelial-like mesothelial cells in their effluent. VEGF production ex vivo by effluent mesothelial cells correlated with serum VEGF level. In addition, Cr-MTC correlated with VEGF levels in culture and serum. Cr-MTC also was associated with mesothelial cell phenotype. VEGF expression in stromal cells, retaining mesothelial markers, was observed in peritoneal biopsy specimens from high-transporter patients. These results suggest that mesothelial cells that have undergone epithelial-to-mesenchymal transition are the main source of VEGF in PD patients and therefore may be responsible for a high peritoneal transport rate [3].

In a clinical study performed by our group, we studied the peritoneal anatomical changes during the first months on PD, and to correlate them with peritoneal functional parameters. We studied 35 stable PD patients for up to 2 years on PD, with a mean age of 45.37 years. Seventy-four percent of patients presented loss of the mesothelial layer, 46% fibrosis and 17% in situ evidence of MMT (submesothelial cytokeratin staining), which increased over time. All patients with MMT showed myofibroblasts, while only 36% of patients without MMT had myofibroblasts. The myofibroblasts represent a dynamic population of cells showing functional and phenotypic diversity. During the last years, numerous different molecules have been reported to be expressed by tissue fibroblasts including peritoneal ones [10]. The origin of tissue fibroblasts has been largely overlooked, so that their lineage is not fully elucidated. There is now evidence supporting that fibro-myofibroblasts might originate from different sources. Firstly, they may differentiate from resident tissue stem cells or fibroblasts. Secondly, they can originate from nearby epithelial cells through a process known as MMT. Finally, the bone marrow and circulating cells may be responsible for the production of fibro-myofibroblasts circulating in the blood stream to their final tissue destination [33].

In PD, emergent evidence points that fibroblasts may arise from local conversion of epithelial cells by MMT or from CD34 + cells (fibrocytes) of the bloodstream after being recruited from bone marrow. In the case of renal fibrosis models, it has been shown that 36% of new fibroblasts derive from MMT, 15% from bone marrow and the rest comes from local proliferation of resident fibroblasts. In PD-related fibrosis, we have demonstrated the expression of mesothelial markers in stromal spindle-like cells, suggesting that they stemmed from local conversion of MC. In contrast, we did not observe a significant contribution of CD34+ cells from bone marrow to the submesothelial fibroblast population in the fibrotic peritoneal tissue [33].

In regard to angiogenesis, the number of peritoneal vessels did not vary when we compared different times on PD. Vasculopathy was present in 17% of the samples. Functional studies were used to define the peritoneal transport status. Patients in the highest quartile of mass transfer area coefficient of creatinine (Cr-MTAC) showed significantly higher MMT prevalence but similar number of peritoneal vessels. In the multivariate analysis, the highest quartile of Cr-MTAC remained as an independent factor predicting the presence of MMT after adjusting for fibrosis [34]. These findings indicate that MMT is a frequent morphological change in the peritoneal membrane. These myofibroblastic cells with submesothelial localization may arise from local conversion of MC during the repair responses and the high solute transport status is associated with MMT.

5. Are MMT, SPS and EPS part of the same process?

From MMT to SPS. Peritoneal fibrosis (or sclerosis) is a term that comprises a wide spectrum of peritoneal structural alterations, ranging from mild inflammation to severe sclerosing peritonitis and its most complicated manifestation, encapsulating peritonitis sclerosis (EPS) [6, 35, 36]. Simple sclerosis (SS), an intermediate stage of peritoneal fibrosis, is the most common peritoneal lesion found in the patients after few months on PD, and could represent the initial phase of sclerosing peritonitis syndrome (SPS). Rubin et al [5] described a normal thickness of the peritoneum of 20 μm, but after a few months on PD could reach up to 40 μm (SS). The SP is a progressive sclerosis that is characterized by a dramatic thickening of the peritoneum (up to 4000 μm) and is accompanied by inflammatory infiltrates, calcification, neo-vascularization and dilatation of blood and lymphatic vessels, being the thickening the most commonly used pathological criterion for differential diagnosis [6, 35, 36].

The importance of establishing a connection between MMT, SPS and EPS is the potential therapeutic and preventive effect of blocking this axis. Also emerging evidence suggests that partial or total blockage of the MMT prevents early stages of PM fibrosis and angiogenesis and preserves the PM function. Moreover, current studies show TGF-β is probably the most important molecule in the PM failure development, so act on a single molecule, the TGF-β, facilitates therapeutic approach. In fact we have shown that blockade of TGF-β significantly attenuated PM failure induced by PD fluids.

One of the biggest problems to establish the definitive connection between SPS and EPS is that the EPS animal model has not been fully and properly developed. While in our mice PD model in 4 or more weeks reaches the typical changes induced by PD fluids on humans, the peritoneal fibrosis model with chlorhexidine results artificial and extremely aggressive. The experimental development of an appropriate EPS model is mandatory. Possibly the most appropriate EPS mice model would be to maintain long-term (months) in PD according to our model of SPS. Once accepted this limitation, the current data suggest that MMT and SPS are part of the process. We have analyzed serially PM pieces of mice in PD at baseline, 15 and 30 days and we found a linear correlation between time on PD, the thickness of the PM and the number of MCs cytokeratin (+) and FSP-1 (+) in the area submesothelial. This phenomenon was accompanied by progressive loss of the mesothelial monolayer which indicates an important participation of the MMT in the development of peritoneal fibrosis (our unpublished results). Using a TGF-β adenovirus model, we found early MMT at 4 day after stimuli intraperitoneal injection that was correlated with PM fibrosis [14]. Similar finding was found by others [15]. Clinically, in MCs serially isolated and cultured from PD effluents, the MMT was present progressively over time in PD and is associated with solute transport disorders and ultrafiltration failure [37]. In PM biopsies from 35 PD stable patients performed during the first 2 years on PD, we demonstrated that the first morphological change in peritoneum that appears as a consequence of PD is submesothelial thickening partially caused by the MMT. This phenotype change is associated with an increase in peritoneal solute transport independent of the number of capillaries present in the tissue [1, 3]. Reaching this point, the following questions arise, as follows: could have peritoneal fibrosis without MMT?, or more specifically, could have MMT without the participation of TGF-β?. Experimental data by us [14] and others [15] indicate that blocking MMT in different degrees result in a significantly attenuation of structural and functional changes of PM. Using the adenovirus (TGF-β) and our PD mice model, the double submesothelial staining for cytokeratin (+) and FSP1 (+) was positive in approximately 37% of activated fibroblasts, indicating its epithelial origin [14]. However, the peritoneal fibrosis is inhibited in more than 50% indicating that direct inhibition of TGF-β with anti-TGF-β peptides inhibited other effects of this molecule as the activation of regional fibroblasts. Promising results have also obtained acting on immune system [38], on AGEs accumulation [39] or on renin-angiotensin system (ACE, AR-II, Paricalcitol) and BMP-7 which also modulate directly or indirectly the TGF-β [40]. These arguments lead us to conclude that TGF-β is a key in the initiation and possibly perpetuation of an uncontrolled MMT, which leads to fibrosis and SPS.

From SPS to EPS. The next question is as follows: at which point the SPS becomes an irreversible process to become EPS? The "two-hit" hypothesis explains the EPS as the result of the PD injury. Two factors are required for the onset of EPS: a predisposing factor, such as peritoneal deterioration from persistent injury caused by peritoneal dialysis (the first "hit"), and an initiating factor, such as inflammatory stimuli superimposed on the chronically injured peritoneum (the second "hit"). Peritoneal deterioration (consisting of mesothelial denudation, interstitial fibrosis, vasculopathy, and angiogenesis) leads to an increased tendency toward plasma exudations that contain fibrin and coagulation factors. The fibrins in the exudates contribute to the intestinal adhesions and formation of fibrin capsule. Inflammatory stimuli caused by infectious peritonitis are superimposed on the damaged peritoneum and act as an initiating factor to trigger the onset of EPS. Inflammatory cytokines also induce activation and proliferation of the peritoneal fibroblasts, promoting peritoneal fibrosis and intestinal adhesions. The relationship between the extent of the first and second "hits" can be demonstrated. The extent of peritoneal damage (the first "hit") increases with the duration of peritoneal dialysis [41, 42].

The onset of EPS depends on the total intensity of both lesions: peritoneal damage and inflammatory stimuli. For the onset of EPS, the total intensity must be greater than a given threshold. The extent of the inflammatory stimuli (the second "hit") are required for the onset of EPS [41, 42].

In both cases (acute and chronic peritoneal injury), the TGF-β is activated with subsequent initiation and perpetuation of MMT and its deleterious effects (fibrosis, angiogenesis, etc.). However, it is very difficult to establish the point of no return in peritoneal lesions clinically because patients with type-I PM failure usually recover functionality and possibly tissue damage with rest peritoneal [43]. In experimental animals, data about fibrosis reversibility are not available. Unfortunately, the initial degree of PM fibrosis has been determined in very few cases (peritoneal biopsies not available). Finally a genetic component cannot be ruled [44, 45].

From MMT to EPS. In both, experimental animals [14, 46] and human peritoneal biopsies from patients within 2 years in PD [34], it seems clear that MMT is an early phenomenon able to determine the degree of peritoneal fibrosis and the future of the PM. But no information about MMT in patients with long term in PD or diagnosis of EPS is available. It is possible that MMT may be an initial phenomenon and few signs of it are in severe stages of fibrosis. However, in bridles and postsurgical adhesions, we have found MMT signs (unpublished data by us), and Bowel adherences may represent an intermediate degree between the SPS and EPS (our unpublished data by us), which encourages to conduct studies aimed to find MMT peritoneum with EPS.

These findings represent important evidence linking both processes, but indirect evidence may also be marked. In human studies [3, 11] and in experimental animals [47], our studies demonstrated a direct relationship between MMT and time on PD. Similarly, the several studies showed a parallel between EPS and time on PD [2, 48]. Another important fact is that peritoneal function studies also show a parallel between high frequency ofMMT ofMCs, high Cr-MTC, and low ultrafiltration. Indeed we observed a higher frequency of mesothelial fibroblastoid phenotype in patients with type Cr-MTC >11 mL/min [3]. Furthermore, as is well known, patients with EPS even displayed these with SPS showed similar functional PM deterioration [35, 49, 50]. Another indirect association between these two events is peritonitis. Yañez-Mo and coworkers [11] found that the frequency of nonepithelioidMCwas associated with episodes of peritonitis, thismeans that peritonitis leads to theMMT. In the case of theEPS, there are some studies in the literature that correlate it with peritonitis events. Previous studies suggest that peritonitis may predispose to EPS, especially if this is caused by *Staphylococcus aureus*, fungi, and/or *Pseudomonas* [9, 51]. There is also an association between persistent infections such as tuberculosis peritonitis and EPS [52]. Although peritonitis and EPS are highly associated in several studies it is also known that, especially in a long-term case, EPS may occur without peritonitis. Moreover, patients that have suffered from more events of peritonitis have a higher incidence of MMT and EPS, which suggest again that these processes are related. Finally, we have analyzed more than 10 peritoneal biopsies from patients with EPS where we had found a significant amount of mesothelial cells (CK +) in the peritoneal submesothelial area, which indicates that despite the significant denudation of the peritoneal MCs monolayer.

6. The MMT as therapeutic target

Based on the concept, that MMT, fibrosis and angiogenesis may be part of the same process of peritoneal membrane failure, therapeutic approaches may be addressed to prevent either MMT of the MC or its deleterious effects such as ECM synthesis and/or VEGF production. In this context, *in vitro* and *ex vivo* cultures of MC may be useful for testing pharmacological agents with potential effects on MMT of the MC. Two molecules with expected preventive effect on the MMT of MC are hepatocyte growth factor (HGF) and bone morphogenic protein-7 (BMP-7). It has been demonstrated that these molecules are able to inhibit and reverse MMT and renal fibrosis in animal models. [53-54]. Other strategies that would open new avenues of therapeutic intervention to prevent or reverse MMT of MC may include the inhibition of ILK, RhoA-ROCK or Akt-mediated signaling cascades [25-33, 55]. In this context, the administration of the ROCK inhibitor Y-27632 resulted in suppression of α-SMA expression and renal interstitial fibrosis in a mouse model of ureteral obstruction. [55]

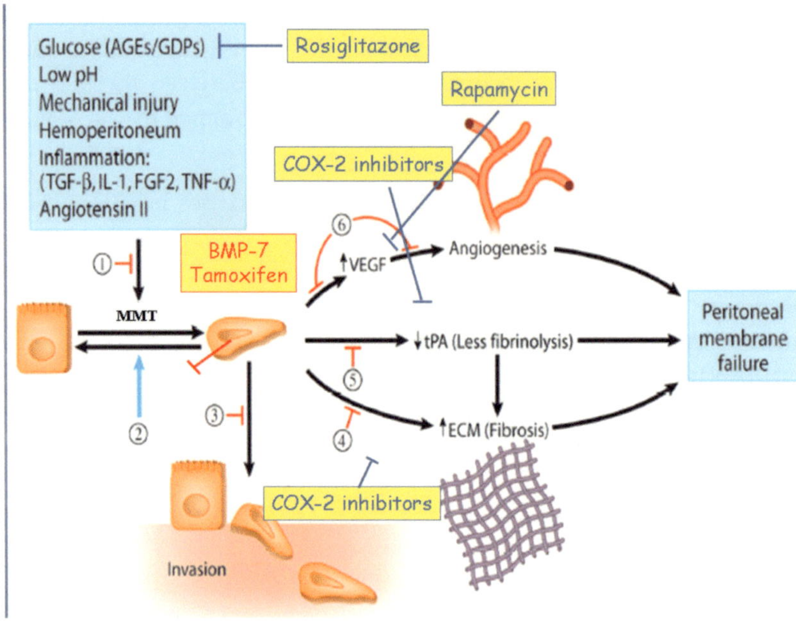

Figure 4. Therapeutic approach to MMT. MMT *in vivo* results from integrated signals that are induced by multiple stimuli. These include elevated glucose and glucose degradation products (GDP) and concentration of PD fluids, which through the formation of advanced glycation-end products (AGE) stimulate the transdifferentiation of MC. The formation of AGE may also be due to the uremic status of the PD patients. The low pH of the dialysates and the mechanical injury during PD fluid exchanges may cause tissue irritation and contribute to chronic inflammation of the peritoneum, which promote MMT. Episodes of bacterial or fungal infections or hemoperitoneum cause acute inflammation and upregulation of cytokines and growth factors such as TGF-β, IL-1, fibroblast growth factor-2 (FGF-2), TNF-α, and angiotensin-II, among others, which are strong inducers of MMT. The therapeutic strategies may be designed either to prevent or to reverse the MMT itself or to treat its effects such as cellular invasion, fibrosis, or angiogenesis. The diagram illustrates six steps related to the MMT process of the MC that can be clinically managed, alone or in combination, to prevent peritoneal membrane failure. The numbers represent the steps where different drugs or molecules can act. 1: Tamoxifen, AGEs accumulation inhibitors (Rosiglitazone), BMP7 and HGF; 2: BMP7 and HGF; 3: Invasion Inhibitors (MMPs blocked); 4: Antifibrotic i, e: rapamycin; 5: Tamoxifen and heparin; 6: Angiogenesis inhibitors (rapamycin, inhinitors CO2, etc.)

We performed our studies using testing different drugs or anti-MMT strategies. We have developed a PD mouse model, this consist in the intra-abdominal catheter implantation with a subcutaneous chamber localized in the top of mouse back. After, we injected a daily intraperitoneal injection of PD solution (1.5-2 mL) at least for 4 weeks. In-vitro we used MCs isolated from omentum and from PD peritoneal effluent. We managed to inhibit the MMT and its adverse effects from using rBMP7 [40]. With Rapamycin got a specific inhibition of fibrosis and the vessels formation specifically lymphatic vessels (56, 57, our unpublished results). Rosiglitazone showed an inhibitory effect on the accumulation of submesothelial AGEs, also anti-inflammatory action mediated by T-cells was observed [39]. Similarly, celecocib inhibited the peritoneal fibrosis by an anti-cox2 effect [38]. MMT also was prevented by tamoxifen. This drug inhibited the peritoneal fibrosis and increased MCs fibrinolytic capacity [47]. Clinically, tamoxifen also improved survival in patients diagnosed of EPS [58]. Paricalcitol acted on smads cascade inhibiting the MMT (our unpublished results). Finally, we were able to inhibit specifically TGF-β with anti-TGF-β specific peptides demonstrating the role of TGF-β in the initiation and perpetuation of MMT [14]. In this context, other promising substances are pentoxifylline, dipyridamole, and emodin [59-61]. Figure 4 summarizes the sites where we may act by blocking the MMT or adverse effects. Some of these drugs and / or therapeutic strategies have been described by our group.

7. Conclusion

Recent findings suggest that in the peritoneum new fibroblast-like cells arise from local conversion of MMT during the repair responses that take place in long-term PD. These trans-differentiated MC may invade the submesothelial tissue and may contribute to peritoneal fibrosis and angiogenesis, which ultimately lead to peritoneal membrane failure. MMT appears as the central point in the pathogenesis of peritoneal damage associated to PD. Current data support a connection between MMT and SPS. However, the jump from SPS to EPS and the connection between MMT and EPS have not been fully established. MMT can be a therapeutic target the blockade of which could benefit especially in initial stages of the process.

Acknowledgements

This work was supported by grant SAF2010-21249 from the "Ministerio de Economia y Competitividad" to M.L.-C. and by grant S2010/BMD-2321 from "Comunidad Autónoma de Madrid" to M.L.-C. and R.S. This work was also partially supported by grants PI 09/0776 from "Fondo de Investigaciones Sanitarias" to A.A. RETICS 06/0016 (REDinREN, Fondos FEDER, EU) to R.S and Baxter Grand nº 10CECEU1008 2010 to AA and ML-C.

Author details

Abelardo Aguilera[1*], Jesús Loureiro[1], Guadalupe Gónzalez-Mateo[2], Rafael Selgas[2] and Manuel López-Cabrera[3]

*Address all correspondence to: abelardo.aguilera@salud.madrid.org aguileraa@terra.es

1 Unidad de Biología Molecular and Servicio de Nefrología. Hospital Universitario de la Princesa, Instituto de Investigación Sanitaria Princesa (IP), Madrid, Spain

2 Hospital Universitario La Paz, Instituto de Investigación Sanitaria la Paz (IdiPAZ), Madrid, Spain

3 Centro de Biología Molecular-Severo Ochoa, CSIC-UAM, Cantoblanco, Madrid, Spain

References

[1] Krediet RT, Lindholm B, Rippe B. Pathophysiology of peritoneal membrane failure. Perit Dial Int Suppl 2000; 20: S22-S42.

[2] Rigby RJ, Hawley CM. Sclerosing peritonitis: The experience in Australia. Nephrol Dial Transplant 1998; 13:154-159.

[3] Aroeira LS, Aguilera A, Selgas R, Ramírez-Huesca M, Pérez-Lozano ML, Cirugeda A, Bajo MA, del Peso G, Sánchez-Tomero JA, Jiménez-Heffernan JA, López-Cabrera M. Mesenchymal conversion of mesothelial cells as a mechanism responsible for high solute transport rate in peritoneal dialysis: role of vascular endothelial growth factor.Am J Kidney Dis 2005; 46: 938-48.

[4] Aguilera A, Yáñez-Mo M, Selgas R, Sánchez-Madrid F, López-Cabrera M. Epithelial to mesenchymal transition as a triggering factor of peritoneal membrane fibrosis and angiogenesis in peritoneal dialysis patients. Curr Opin Investig Drugs. 2005; 6: 262-268.

[5] Rubin J, Herrera GA, Collins D. An autopsy study of peritoneal cavity from patients on continuous ambulatory peritoneal dialysis. Am J Kidney Dis 1991; 18:97-102.

[6] Di Paolo N, Garosi G. Peritoneal sclerosis. J Nephrol 1999; 12:347-361.

[7] Di Paolo N, Sacchi G, Garosi G,Taganelli P, Gaggiotti E. SPS and sclerosing peritonitis: related or distinct entities? Int J Artif Organs 2005;28:117-28.

[8] Nagy JA. Peritoneal membrane morphology and function, Kidney Int Suppl 1996;50: 56: S2-S11.

[9] Gotloib L, Shostak A,Wajsbrot V. Functional structure of peritoneum as dialyzing membrane. In: The text book of peritoneal dialysis, 2nd ed: London: Kluwer Academic Publishers; 2000:37-106.

[10] López-Cabrera M, Aguilera A, Aroeira LS, Ramírez-Huesca M, Pérez-Lozano ML, Jiménez-Heffernan JA, Bajo MA, del Peso G, Sánchez-Tomero JA, Selgas R. Ex vivo analysis of dialysis effluent-derived mesothelial cells as an approach to unveiling the mechanism of peritoneal membrane failure. Perit Dial Int 2006; 26: 26-34

[11] Yáñez-Mó M, Lara-Pezzi E, Selgas R, Ramírez-Huesca M, Domínguez-Jiménez C, Jiménez-Heffernan JA, Aguilera A, Sánchez-Tomero JA, Bajo MA, Alvarez V, Castro MA, del Peso G, Cirujeda A, Gamallo C, Sánchez-Madrid F, López-Cabrera M. Peritoneal dialysis and epithelial-to-mesenchymal transition of mesothelial cells.N Engl J Med 2003; 348: 403-413.

[12] Aroeira LS, Aguilera A, Sánchez-Tomero JA, Bajo MA, del Peso G, Jiménez-Heffernan JA, Selgas R, López-Cabrera M. Epithelial to mesenchymal transition and perito-

neal membrane failure in peritoneal dialysis patients: pathologic significance and potential therapeutic interventions. J Am Soc Nephrol 2007; 18: 2004-2013.

[13] Freser D, Wakefield L, Phillips A. Independent regulation of transforming growth factor beta 1 transcription and translation by glucose and platelet-derived growth factor. Am J Pathol 2002; 161: 1039-1049.

[14] Loureiro J, Aguilera A, Selgas R, Sandoval P, Albar-Vizcaíno P, Pérez-Lozano ML, Ruiz-Carpio V, Majano PL, Lamas S, Rodríguez-Pascual F, Borras-Cuesta F, Dotor J, López-Cabrera M. Blocking TGF-β1 protects the peritoneal membrane from dialysate-induced damage. J Am Soc Nephrol. 2011; 22: 1682-95.

[15] Margetts PJ, Kolb M, Hoff CM, Gauldie J. The role of angiopoietins in resolution of angiogenesis resulting from adenoviral mediated gene transfer of TGF-β1 or VEGF to the rat peritoneum. J Am Soc Nephrol. 2001; 12: 2029-2039.

[16] Border WA, Noble NA. Transforming growth factor β in tissue fibrosis. N Engl J Med 1994; 331: 1286-1292.

[17] Massagué J, Wotton D. Transcriptional control by the TGF-β/Smad signaling. EMBO 2000; 19: 1745-1754.

[18] Fan JM, Ng YY, Hill PA, Nikolic-Paterson DJ, Mu W, Atkins RC, Lan HY. Transforming growth factor-beta regulate tubular epithelial-myofibroblast transdifferenciation in vitro. Kidney Int 1999; 56: 1455-1467.

[19] Tan C, Mui A, Dedhar S. Integrin-linked kinase regulate inducible nitric oxide synthase and cyclooxygenase-2 expression in an NF-κB-dependent manner. J Biol Chem 2002; 277: 3109-3116.

[20] Bitzer M, Von Gersdorff G, Liang D, Dominguez-Rosales A, Beg AA, Rojkind M, Böttinger EP. A mechanism of supression of TGF-β/SMAD signalling by NF-κB/Re1A. Genes and Development 2000; 14: 187-197.

[21] Cano A, Pérez-Moreno MA, Rodrigo I, Locascio A, Blanco MJ, del Barrio MG, Portillo F, Nieto MA. The transcription factor snail controls epithelial-mesenchymal transitions by repressing E-cadherin expression. Nat Cell Biol 2000; 2: 76-83.

[22] Poser I, Dominguez D, de Herreros AG, Varnai A, Buettner R, Bosserhoff AK. Loss of E-cadherin expression in melanoma cells involves up-regulation of the transcriptional repressor Snail. J Biol Chem 2001; 276: 24661-24666.

[23] Vega S, Morales AV, Ocaña OH, Valdés F, Fabregat I, Nieto MA. Snail blocks the cell cycle and confers resistance to cell death. Genes and Development 2004; 18: 1131-1143.

[24] D'Amico M, Hulit J, Amanatullah DF, Zafonte BT, Albanese C, Bouzahzah B, Fu M, Augenlicht LH, Donehower LA, Takemaru K, Moon RT, Davis R, Lisanti MP, Shtutman M, Zhurinsky J, Ben-Ze'ev A, Troussard AA, Dedhar S, Pestell RG. The integrin-linked kinase regulates the cyclin D1 gene through glycogen synthase kinase 3β and

cAM-responsive element-binding protein-dependent pathways. J Biol Chem 2000; 275: 32649-32657.

[25] Kim K, Lu Z, Hay ED. Direct evidence for a role of beta-catenin/LEF-1 signaling pathway in induction of EMT. Cell Biol Int 2002; 26: 463-476.

[26] Troussard AA, Costello P, Yoganathan TN, Kumagai S, Roskelley CD, Dedhar S. The integrin linked kinase (ILK) induces an invasive phenotype via AP-1 transcription factor-dependent upregulation of matrix metalloproteinase 9 (MMP-9). Oncogene 2000; 16: 5444-5452.

[27] Masszi A, Di Ciano, Sirokmany G, Arthur WT, Rotstein OD, Wang J, McCulloch CA, Rosivall L, Mucsi I, Kapus A. Central role for Rho in TGF-beta1-induced alpha-smooth muscle actin expresion during epithelial-mesenchymal transition. Am J Physiol Renal Physiol 2003; 284:F911-F924.

[28] Benitah SA, Valeron PF, Lacal JC. ROCK and nuclear factor-kappaB-dependent activation of cyclooxygenase-2 by Rho GTPases: Effects on tumor growth and therapeutic consequences. Mol Biol Cell 2003; 14: 3041-3054.

[29] Huber MA, Azoitei N, Baumann B, Grünert S, Sommer A, Pehamberger H, Kraut N, Beug H, Wirth T. NF-κB is essential for epithelial-mesenchymal transition and metastasis in a model of breast cancer progression. J Clin Invest 2004; 114:569-581.

[30] Barberà MJ, Puig I, Domínguez D, Julien-Grille S, Guaita-Esteruelas S, Peiró S, Baulida J, Francí C, Dedhar S, Larue L, García de Herreros A. Regulation of snail transcription during epithelial to mesenchymal transition of tumor cells. Oncogene 2004; 23: 7345-7354.

[31] Peinado H, Quintanilla M, Cano A. Transforming growth factor β-1 induces snail transcription factor in epithelial cell lines. J Biol Chem 2003; 278: 21113-21123.

[32] Li Y, Yang J, Dai C, Wu C, Liu Y. Role for intergrin-linked kinase in mediating tubular epithelial to mesenchymal transition and renal interstitial fibrogenesis. J Clin Invest 2003; 112: 503-516.

[33] Del Peso G, Jimenez-Heffernan JA, Bajo MA, Hevia C, Aguilera A, Castro MJ, Sanchez-Tomero JA, Lopez-Cabrera M, Selgas R. Myofibroblastic differentiation in simple peritoneal sclerosis. Int J Artif Organs 2005; 28: 135-140.

[34] Del Peso G, Jiménez-Heffernan JA, Bajo MA, Aroeira LS, Aguilera A, Fernández-Perpén A, Cirugeda A, Castro MJ, de Gracia R, Sánchez-Villanueva R, Sánchez-Tomero JA, López-Cabrera M, Selgas R. Epithelial-to-mesenchymal transition of mesothelial cells is an early event during peritoneal dialysis and is associated with high peritoneal transport. Kidney Int Suppl 2008; 108: S26-33.

[35] Nomoto Y, Kawaguchi Y, Kubo H, Hirano H, Sikai S, Kurokawa K. Sclerosing encapsulanting peritonitis in patients undergoing continuous ambulatory peritoneal dialy-

sis: a report of sclerosing encapsulating peritonitis group. Am J Kidney Dis 1996; 28: 420-427.

[36] Schneble F, Bonzel KE, Waldherr R, Bachmann S, Roth H, Schärer K. Peritoneal morphology in children treated by continuous ambulatory peritoneal dialysis. Pediatr Nephrol 1992; 6: 542-546.

[37] Do JY, Kim YL, Park JW, Chang KA, Lee SH, Ryu DH, Kim CD, Park SH, Yoon KW. The association between the vascular endothelial growth factor-to-cancer antigen 125 ratio in peritoneal dialysis effluent and the epithelial-to-mesenchymal transition in continuous ambulatory peritoneal dialysis. Perit Dial Int Suppl. 2008; 28: S101-S106.

[38] Aroeira LS, Lara-Pezzi E, Loureiro J, Aguilera A, Ramírez-Huesca M, González-Mateo G, Pérez-Lozano ML, Albar-Vizcaíno P, Bajo MA, del Peso G, Sánchez-Tomero JA, Jiménez-Heffernan JA, Selgas R, López-Cabrera M. Cyclooxygenase-2 mediates dialysate-induced alterations of the peritoneal membrane. J Am Soc Nephrol 2009; 20: 582-592.

[39] Sandoval P, Loureiro J, González-Mateo G, Pérez-Lozano ML, Maldonado-Rodríguez A, Sánchez-Tomero JA, Mendoza L, Santamaría B, Ortiz A, Ruíz-Ortega M, Selgas R, Martín P, Sánchez-Madrid F, Aguilera A, López-Cabrera M. PPAR-γ agonist rosiglitazone protects peritoneal membrane from dialysis fluid-induced damage. Lab Invest 2010; 90: 1517-1532

[40] Loureiro J, Schilte M, Aguilera A, Albar-Vizcaíno P, Ramírez-Huesca M, Pérez-Lozano ML, González-Mateo G, Aroeira LS, Selgas R, Mendoza L, Ortiz A, Ruíz-Ortega M, van den Born J, Beelen RH, López-Cabrera M. BMP-7 blocks mesenchymal conversion of mesothelial cells and prevents peritoneal damage induced by dialysis fluid exposure. Nephrol Dial Transplant. 2010; 25: 1098-1108

[41] K. Honda K Oda H, "Pathology of encapsulating peritoneal sclerosis," Perit Dial Int Suppl 2005; 25: S19–S29

[42] Barini G, Schuinski A, Moraes TP, Meyer F, Pecoits-Filho R, "Inflammation and the peritoneal membrane: causes and impact on structure and function during peritoneal dialysis," Mediators Inflamm. 2012; 2012: 912595.

[43] de Alvaro F, Castro MJ, Dapena F, Bajo MA, Fernandez-Reyes MJ, Romero JR, Jimenez C, Miranda B, Selgas R. Peritoneal resting is beneficial in peritoneal hyperpermeability and ultrafiltration failure. Adv Perit Dial. 1993; 9: 56-61.

[44] Gillerot G, Goffin E, Michel C, Evenepoel P, Biesen WV, Tintillier M, Stenvinkel P, Heimbürger O, Lindholm B, Nordfors L, Robert A, Devuyst O. Genetic and clinical factors influence the baseline permeability of the peritoneal membrane. Kidney Int. 2005; 67: 2477–2487.

[45] Numata M, Nakayama M, Hosoya T, Hoff CM, Holmes CJ, Schalling M, Nordfors L, Lindholm B. Possible pathologic involvement of receptor for advanced glycation end

products (RAGE) for development of encapsulating peritoneal sclerosis in Japanese CAPD patients. Clin Nephrol 2004; 62: 455–460.

[46] Margetts PJ, Bonniaud P, Liu L,.Transient overexpression of TGF-β1 induces epithelial mesenchymal transition in the rodent peritoneum. J Am Soc Nephrol 2005; 16: 425–436.

[47] Loureiro J, Sandoval P, del Peso G, Gónzalez-Mateo G, Fernández-Millara V, Bajo MA, Sánchez-Tomero JA, Guerra-Azcona G, Selgas R, López-Cabrera M, Aguilera AI.. Tamoxifen Ameliorates Peritoneal Membrane Damage by Blocking Mesothelial to Mesenchymal Transition in Peritoneal Dialysis. Plos One 2013; 8: e61165.

[48] H. Kawanishi H, Moriishi M. Epidemiology of encapsulating peritoneal sclerosis in Japan. Perit Dial Int Supp 2005; 25, 4: S14–S18.

[49] Kawaguchi Y, Hasegawa T, Kubo H, Yamamoto H, Nakayama M, Shigematsu T. Current issues of continuous ambulatory peritoneal dialysis. Artif Organs, 1995; 19: 1204–1209.

[50] Afthentopoulos IE, Passadakis P, Oreopoulos DG, Bargman J. Erratum: sclerosing peritonitis in continuous ambulatory peritoneal dialysis patients: one center's experience and review of the literature, Adv Ren Repl Ther 1998; 5: 157-167.

[51] Slingeneyer A. Preliminary report on a cooperative international study on sclerosing encapsulating peritonitis. Nephrol Dial Transplant 1988; 3: 66–69.

[52] Bentley PG, Higgs DR. Peritoneal tuberculosis with ureteric obstruction, mimicking retroperitoneal fibrosis. B J Urol 1976; 48: 170-1976.

[53] Yang J, Liu Y. Blockage of tubular epithelial to myofibroblast transition by hepatocyte growth factor prevents renal interstitial fibrosis. J Am Soc Nephrol 2002; 13: 96-207.

[54] Zeisberg M, Hanai J, Sugimoto H, Mammoto T, Charytan D, Strutz F, Kalluri R. BMP-7 counteracts TGF-β1-induced epithelial-to-mesenchymal transition and reverses chronic renal injury. Nat Med 2003; 9: 964-968.

[55] Nagatoya K, Moriyama T, Kawada N, Takeji M, Oseto S, Murozono T, Ando A, Imai E, Hori M. Y-27632 prevents tubulo-interstitial fibrosis in mouse kidneys with unilateral ureteral obstruction. Kidney Int 2002; 61: 1684-1695.

[56] Sekiguchi Y, Zhang J, Patterson S, Liu L, Hamada C, Tomino Y, Margetts PJ. Rapamycin inhibits transforming growth factor β-induced peritoneal angiogenesis by blocking the secondary hypoxic response. J Cell Mol Med. 2012; 16: 1934-45.

[57] Aguilera A, Aroeira LS, Ramirez-Huesca M, Perez-Lozano ML, Cirugeda A, Bajo MA, Del Peso G, Valenzuela-Fernandez A, Sanchez-Tomero JA, Lopez-Cabrera M, Selgas R. Effects of rapamycin on the epithelial-to-mesenchymal transition of human peritoneal mesothelial cells. Int J Artif Organs 2005; 28: 164-169.

[58] del Peso G, Bajo MA, Gil F, Aguilera A, Ros S, Costero O, Castro MJ, Selgas R. Clinical experience with tamoxifen in peritoneal fibrosing syndromes. Adv Perit Dial 2003; 19: 32-35.

[59] Fang CC, Yen CJ, Chen YM, Shyu RS, Tsai TJ, Lee PH, Hsieh BS. Pentoxifylline inhibits human peritoneal mesothelail cell growth and collagen synthesis: Effects in TGF-β. Kidney Int 2000; 57: 2626-2633.

[60] Hung KY, Chen CT, Huang JW, Lee PH, Tsai TJ, Hsieh BS. Dipyrodamole inhibits TGF-beta-induced collagen gene expression in human peritoneal mesothelial cells. Kidney Int 2001; 60: 1249-1257.

[61] Chan TM, Leung JK, Tsang RC, Liu ZH, Li LS, Yung S. Emodin ameliorates glucose-induced matrix synthesis in human peritoneal mesothelial cells. Kidney Int 2003; 64:519-533.

Chapter 3

Encapsulating Peritoneal Sclerosis

Joerg Latus, Christoph Ulmer, Martin Kimmel,
M. Dominik Alscher and Niko Braun

Additional information is available at the end of the chapter

http://dx.doi.org/10.5772/56052

1. Introduction

Chronic peritoneal dialysis (PD) can be complicated by encapsulating peritoneal sclerosis (EPS), a rare but the most severe complication associated with long-term PD. Morbidity and mortality are still high (range from 25% to 55%) especially in the first year after diagnosis. The international Society for Peritoneal Dialysis (ISPD) defined EPS by clinical signs of abdominal pain, bowel obstruction or weight loss in late stages of the disease. Clinical symptoms, radiologic findings and histologic criteria are the three diagnostic pillars.

During the course of the disease, development of adhesions causing symptoms of bowel obstruction often requires major surgery (figure 1A). Mostly, peritonectomy and enterolysis (PEEL) is the surgical treatment of choice.

Earlier stages of the disease are difficult to detect. Changes in transporter status or ultrafiltration failure can be first signs of EPS. The incidence of EPS increases with increasing time on PD, younger age, glucose load and peritonitis rate. EPS may occur when the patient is still on PD, but most patients become symptomatic after cessation of PD. In the minority of cases, EPS symptoms disappear and it seems to be a selflimiting condition. Actually, there exist no evidence based medical and surgical treatment options. Case reports and small case series are dealing with the effectiveness of immunosuppressants or antifibrotic drugs. But evidence for a specific medical treatment option is still lacking and prospective studies are needed.

2. Epidemiology of encapsulating peritoneal sclerosis

EPS is a very rare disease and the true incidence is still unknown. It is not exclusively seen in patients on PD but in this chapter we will focus only on PD-patients or former PD-patients.

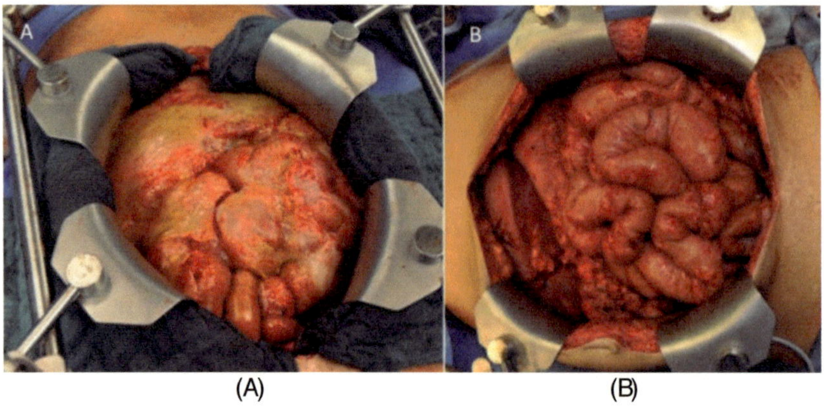

Figure 1. A 45-year old male presenting with massive abdominal pain, nausea, vomiting and weight loss over months. He was on PD for 72 months. EPS shows a sticky fibrin coating membrane on top of the bowel containing the brown and thick peritoneum B After an operation time of 420 minutes with peritonectomy and enterolysis (PEEL). Fibrin membranes were resected and restitution of intestinal function was achieved. 72 months after surgery, he has completely recovered and is back at work.

Kawanishi et al. reported 2004 and 2005 in their large cohorts, an overall incidence of 2.5% with an even higher incidence of up to 17.2% for patients on PD longer than 15 years. The Scottish Renal Registry included 1238 PD patients and Brown et al. showed that the incidence of EPS increases with time on PD: 2% after three to four years, 8.8% after five to six years and 5% after more than six years on PD. Interestingly, at the time of EPS diagnosis, 26% of the patients were still on PD whereas 72% were not on PD. Recently, Johnson et al. showed in a very large study from Australia and New Zealand a remarkably low incidence of 0.3, 0.8 and 3.9% after three, five and eight years on PD. In this study, the hazard ratio for patients receiving more than eight years PD was 12.1 in this study. It is noteworthy, that all existing data indicate that the majority of patients who are on PD for a long time will not develop EPS. The probability to develop e.g. endocarditis or osteomyelitis is much higher. Nevertheless, several risk factors for the development of EPS are discussed, but the published data are not uniform (table 1).

3. Diagnostic pillars in encapsulating peritoneal sclerosis

3.1. Clinical features of encapsulating peritoneal sclerosis

The clinical features of EPS are the result of acute or subacute small bowel obstruction mostly caused by adhesions and signs of systemic inflammation. The clinical findings mostly seen in patients with EPS are summarized in Table 2. In one of our EPS studies, all patients in the severe group (which was defined by the requirement for surgery due to extensive symptoms caused by bowel obstruction) had massive abdominal pain or vomiting. A large proportion in this group had both symptoms. Additionally, weight loss was noted in almost all patients in this group. In earlier stages of the disease, loss of peritoneal ultrafiltration capacity with weight gain (9 out of 31 in our study), a lower residual renal function, a higher glucose and icodextrin

http://dx.doi.org/10.5772/56052

Longer duration of PD
High Peritonitis Rate (severity/staphylococcus aureus)
High Glucose Exposure
Ultrafiltration failure
High volume regimen
Absence of residual renal function
Inadequate dialysis (low Kt/V)
Younger age
Cessation of PD (post-transplant)
Acetate buffer
Chlorhexidine
Icodextrin use
Medication (ß-Blocker, calcineurin inhibitors)
Smoking status

Table 1. Possible risk factors for EPS (most confident risk factors are marked in bold)

exposure are common. High transporter status in the peritoneal equilibration test prior to development of EPS has also been described in many EPS patients. These membrane changes are, however, not indicative for EPS, because they are also commonly observed in patients on long-term PD who do not develop EPS. Japanese investigators made an approach to subcategorize EPS in four stages. The first stage means the so-called pre-EPS stage with ascites followed by an inflammatory stage. Third stage is a stage of encapsulating of the bowel and the final stage includes symptoms of bowel obstruction. Up to now, this staging is not widely accepted in the international PD community.

Symptoms and clinical findings in EPS patients	
Signs of bowel obstruction	Signs of Inflammation
• Appetite loss	• Fever
• Nausea and vomiting	• Ascites
• Abdominal pain	• General fatigue
• Abdominal fullness	• Weight loss
• Diarrhea	Peritoneal adhesions
• Anorexia	• Bloody effluent
• Weight loss	• Ascites
• Feeling of heaviness	• Abdominal pain
• Constipation	• Abdominal mass
• Absent bowel sounds	

Table 2. Common clinical findings in patients EPS

3.2. Radiological findings in encapsulating peritoneal sclerosis

A CT-scan is mandatory in all patients with suspected EPS, but it is noteworthy, that no single diagnostic feature on CT-scan exists and any of the mentioned features can be found in scans of PD-patients without EPS. There is rarely more than one feature and in the majority of cases of low severity. Therefore, current evidence does not support the use of CT scanning to screen for EPS. Table 3 summarizes the typical imaging features of EPS and figure 2 shows an example of a 59-year old male with late-stage EPS. In very rare cases, x-rays show massive calcification (figure 3). Other studies like ultrasound, MRI or abdominal X-ray are insufficiently sensitive, rarely typical features are found.

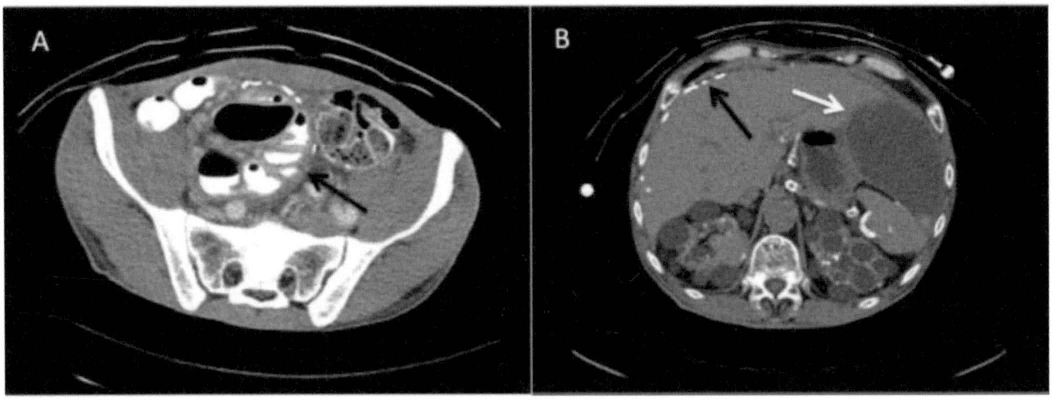

Figure 2. A CT scan showing typical „cocooning" with heavy calcifications and bowel obstruction (arrow). B Thickening, calcification and enhancement of the peritoneal membrane (black arrow). Loculated fluid collection (white arrow).

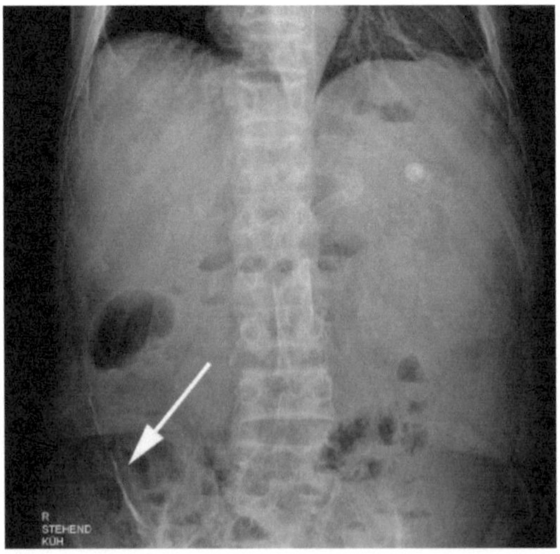

Figure 3. Peritoneal calcification (arrow) in a patient with established EPS after 22 years on PD.

http://dx.doi.org/10.5772/56052

Adhesion of bowel loops
Peritoneal thickening
Peritoneal calcification
Peritoneal enhancement
Bowel dilatation
Change of bowel calibre
Fluid loculation/septation
Thickening of the bowel wall

Table 3. Computed tomographic findings of EPS patients

3.3. Histological criteria for encapsulating peritoneal sclerosis

The third diagnostic pillar of EPS is based on the evaluation of peritoneal biopsies. The diagnosis of PD-associated pathologies, especially of EPS, is an interdisciplinary process, which requires, nephrologists and pathologists. The two most relevant pathologies of long-term PD are simple sclerosis (SS), which is a very common finding in PD- and EPS- patients. For a histological diagnosis, reproducible histological criteria are needed that can be used to differentiate the two entities. In 2003 and 2005 Honda and colleagues investigated peritoneal biopsies of 12 EPS patients. Fibrin deposition, fibroblast swelling, capillary angiogenesis and mononuclear cell infiltration were significantly more common in EPS than in peritonitis, ultrafiltration failure, uremia and so called "pre-EPS". Regarding the degree of these parameters, only fibroblast swelling and fibrin deposition exhibited were statistically significant different in their study. Several markers for fibroblast proliferation were also investigated. Garosi and colleagues investigated 224 peritoneal biopsies of non-EPS patients and compared the morphological findings with the biopsies of 39 patients with EPS. Significant findings in patients with EPS were thickening of the submesothelial cell layer, vasculopathy, arterial occlusion, inflammation, tissue calcification and ossification and arterial calcification and ossification (figure 4). In 2008 Sherif and colleagues compared peritoneal biopsies of 12 EPS patients with 23 non-EPS patients. Only fibrin deposition and the thickness of the compacta were significantly different between EPS patients and non-EPS patients. Actually, there is one main problem associated with most of the published data. In these previous studies, data acquisition was not standardized, observers were not blinded to the diagnosis and intra- and inter-observer variability was not given. Up to now there is no established method to differentiate between EPS and simple sclerosis. Especially in this field, further studies are needed to establish standardized histological criteria for EPS.

4. Pathogenic models of encapsulating peritoneal sclerosis

4.1. Epithelio-mesenchymal transformation (EMT) and the so-called two-hit-model

Over the years, the non-physiological properties of the PD fluids (glucose load, acidic pH, GDP`s affects the integrity of the peritoneal membrane. The insult of the serosa leads to

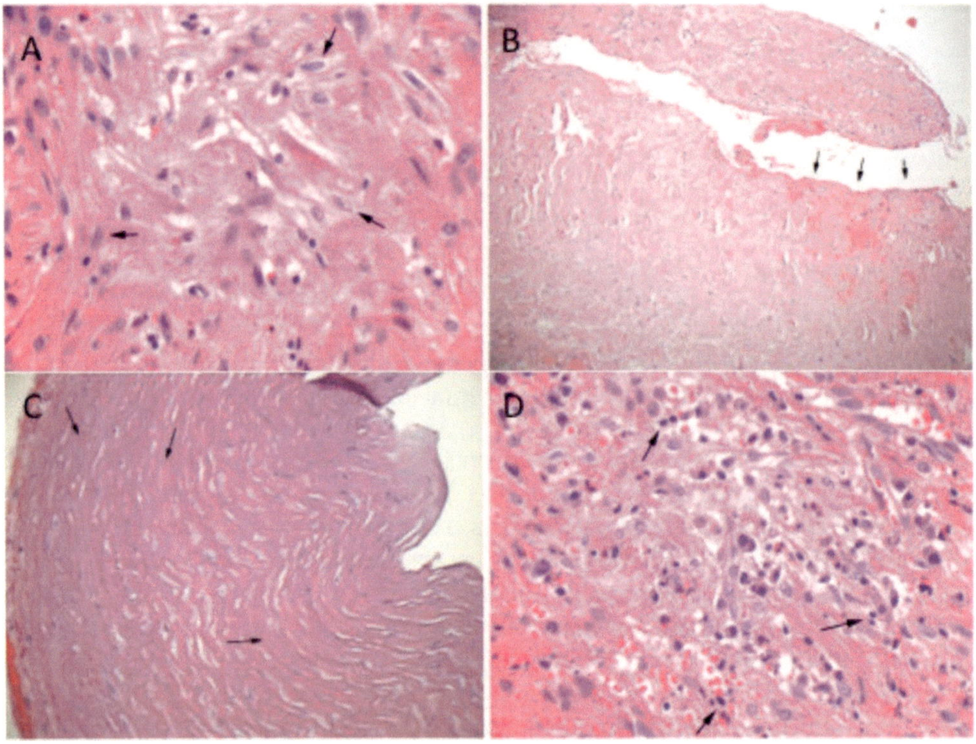

Figure 4. Peritoneal biopsies of EPS patients A HE staining showing an increased cellularity, round cells and fibroblast like cells (arrows). EPS, original magnification x400 B HE staining showing a decreased cellularity, fibrin deposits and a complete denudation of the mesothelial cell layer with fibrin exudations (arrows). EPS, original magnification x100 C HE staining showing a decreased cellularity with intracellular matrix (arrows), complete mesothelial denudation with fibrin exudations. EPS, original magnification x200 D HE staining showing fibroblast like cells, eosinophils, plasma cells and round cells (arrows). EPS, original magnification x400

secretion and production of different profibrinogenic mediators like transforming growth factor (TGF)-ß and of angiogenic factors like vascular endothelial growth factor (VEGF). The profibrinogenic factors lead to an increased fibrin deposition and neoangiogenesis. Additionally, the degradation of fibrin is reduced due to the loss of mesothelial cells and mast cells, which under normal circumstances produce fibrinolytic substances. This results in a so-called epithelio-mesenchymal transformation (EMT) (figure 5). As a consequence mesothelial cells change their function and become a more myofibroblast-like phenotype, which leads to the deposition of extracellular matrix and the promotion of fibrosis (figure 5). The described mechanisms lead to peritoneal fibrosis (PF), but do not necessarily proceed to EPS.

In the so-called two-hit-model of the pathogenesis of simple peritoneal fibrosis (PF) and EPS, it is postulated that PD itself is the first hit leading to the damage of the peritoneal membrane. When the second hit (e.g. an inflammatory stimulus (like a bacterial peritonitis)) occurs, EPS can develop. Others state, that EPS occurs in every patient on PD depending on the time on PD. Peritonitis rates, glucose load of the PD solutions and other factors might only influence this process.

http://dx.doi.org/10.5772/56052

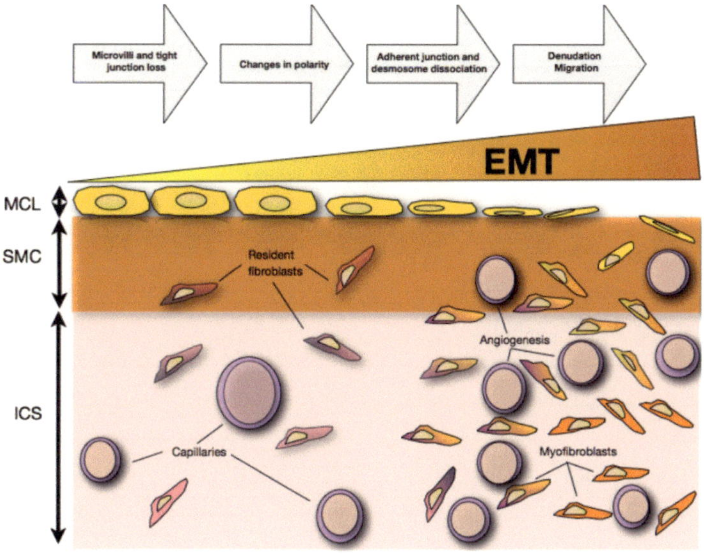

Figure 5. Mesothelial cells undergoing the so-called epithelio-mesenchymal transformation (EMT); MCL mesothelial cell layer; SMC sub mesothelial cells; ICS interstitial cell space. Adapted from Aroeira et al..

5. Management and outcome in encapsulating peritoneal sclerosis

The optimal management of EPS is not clear. Mortality and morbidity are still high (25% to 55%) especially in the first year after diagnosis. Table 4 shows a comparison of epidemiological studies of EPS patients. Up to now, there are no randomized controlled trials and the level of evidence is weak. The choice of surgical or conservative therapy is often based on the stage of the disease and varies quiet a lot between "EPS- centers". There is one prospective registry report from Kawanishi et al., who investigated 48 EPS patients in Japan. They report a recovery rate with total parenteral nutrition, corticosteroids and surgical treatment of 0%, 38.5% and 58.3%, respectively. All together, 37.5% of the patients in this study died, 45.8% of the patients recovered.

During work-up of patients with EPS, bacterial and fungal peritonitis must be ruled out before treatment might be considered. Treatment options include surgery and/or medical therapy.

5.1. Medical therapy

Steroids: Data about the use of steroids are not uniform, especially concerning dose and duration of therapy. Some studies suggested the administration of methylprednisolone pulse therapy with a dose of 500 – 1000 mg daily for 2-3 days, resulting in a reduction of inflammation and improvement of symptoms of bowel obstruction. Other groups recommend a dose of 0.5–1mg prednisolone per kilogram of body weight daily for 2-4 weeks. In our referral- center we recommend an initial dose of 1 mg prednisolone per kilogram body weight for 4 weeks,

	Date of study	EPS cases	Study design	Mean PD duration (years)	Mortality rate (%)
Nomoto et al. (Japan 1996)	1980-1994	62	RS/MC	5.1	43.5
Rigby et al. (Australia 1998)	1980-1994	54	RS/MC	4.3	56
Lee et al. (Korea 2003)	1981-2002	31	RS/MC	5.8	25.8
Kawanishi et al. (Japan 2001)	1999-2001	17	PS/MC	10	35
Kawanishi et al. (Japan 2004)	1999-2003	48	PS/MC	4.3	37.5
Summers et al. (UK 2005)	1998-2003	27	RS/SC	6.1	29.6
Brown et al. (UK 2009)	2000-2007	46	RS/MC	5.4	56.5
Balasubramaniam et al. (UK 2009)	1997-2008	111	RS/MC	6.9	53
Johnson et al. (Australia 2010)	1995-2007	33	RS/MC	4.5	55
Kawanishi et al. (Japan 2011)	1993-2010	181	RS/MC	10.5	35.4
Latus et al. (Germany 2012)	1998-2011	42	RS/SC	6.5	21.4

Table 4. Comparison of epidemiological studies of EPS; RS, retrospective; PS, prospective; MC, multi-center; SC, single-center;

followed by a slow tapering over months depending on clinical symptoms and signs of inflammation. Especially in the so-called inflammatory period of the disease steroids may be useful. A prospective study demonstrated clinical improvement in 35.7% of cases treated with prednisolone. In patients with late-stage disease, histological analysis of peritoneal biopsies showed less acute or chronic inflammation. Therefore, the use of steroids is questionable.

Immunosuppression: The present evidence for the use of immunosuppressants (e.g. mycophenolate or azathioprine) is mainly based on case reports. An increasing number of post-transplant EPS has been reported. One reason for the development of post-transplant EPS could be the widespread use of calcineurin inhibitors and the profibrotic potential of these drugs.

Antifibrotic agents: Several different antifibrotic agents are currently under investigation concerning development of peritoneal fibrosis and EPS. In animal models, inhibition of the renin-angiotensin-aldosterone system (RAAS) results in a decreased progression of peritoneal fibrosis. In induced EPS in rats, the blockage of RAAS resulted in a decrease of neoangiogenesis, peritoneal thickening and ultrafiltration failure. Up to now, there exist no data regarding the use of angiotensin receptor blockers (ARB) or angiotensin converting enzyme (ACE) inhibitors in patients with EPS. But due to the low rate of adverse events and the widespread use of this medication in PD patients, inhibition of the RAAS should be the cornerstone of prevention of simple sclerosis and EPS. Tamoxifen, another antifibrotic drug, commonly used in the treatment of breast cancer, has been investigated in EPS patients. Tamoxifen revealed positive results in other fibrosing syndromes such as retroperitoneal fibrosis, fibrosing mediastinitis or desmoid tumors. Individual case reports and small case series supported the use of tamoxifen in EPS patients, mostly in combination with corticosteroids or as monotherapy. Recently, Korte and colleagues demonstrated in a retrospective analysis a survival advantage for patients with EPS treated with tamoxifen. Of the well-matched 63 patients with EPS, 24 were treated with tamoxifen and 39 were not. The mortality rate was significantly reduced in the tamoxifen group compared to the non-tamoxifen group (45.8% vs. 74.4%). The exact mechanism of action of tamoxifen in EPS is not understood. Some data suggest that an enhancement of transforming growth factor-ß (TGF-ß1) production stimulates metalloproteinase-9 to degrade type IV collagen. Other studies demonstrated an overexpression of TGF-ß1 which promoted fibrosis, peritoneal thickening and a loss of the capability of peritoneal repair. Therefore one mechanism of action of tamoxifen could be the inhibition of TGF. Other reports about the use of antifibrotic drugs like cholchicine or pirfenidone did not achieve acceptance in the PD community.

If medical therapy fails to improve the symptoms of EPS, surgical therapy must be considered.

5.2. Surgical therapy

Most data of operative treatment of EPS involve only small series or case reports. Macroscopically, late-stage EPS consists of two layers: a grossly thickened, leather-like peritoneum (EPS-membrane) and a white and opaque EPS-capsule covering the whole abdominal cavity. In contrast to the first description of the disease by Winne et al., EPS-capsule is the result of a dynamic process of shrinking. As a consequence, stricturing of the small bowel, sclerotic loop-to-loop adhesions and severe kinking of multiple bowel loops occur, causing symptoms of small bowel obstruction.

Although associated with a high morbidity and mortality rate, operative treatment probably represents the only realistic and potentially curative treatment for patients with late-stage disease. Because EPS is a rare disease, not all surgeons are familiar with the natural history of EPS and the required operative therapy. EPS is a disease of the visceral peritoneum and the serosa. Therefore, the operative treatment involves a complex procedure comprising *peritonectomy and intestinal enterolysis* (PEEL). Basic requirements of PEEL are the restitution of intestinal function and the prevention of recurrent disease. Simple adhesiolysis is not the treatment of choice. In fact, PEEL includes a demanding resection of EPS-capsule and EPS-membrane, whereas a partial resection of the small bowel serosa is unavoidable. Resection lines often involve the serosa or are located between the serosa and muscularis. With an incidence up to 20%, fistulas or anastomotic leaks are the leading complications after PEEL. Regarding this high morbidity rate, some authors suggest a protective stoma proximal to the first suture of bowel wall defects or anastomoses. Recently, we reviewed the treatment of 26 late-stage EPS patients at our referral center regarding perioperative morbidity, mortality, and long term outcome. In our study, overall morbidity was 44% with minor complications in 2 patients (7%) and major complications in 11 patients (31%). Three patients (10%) died within the first year after operative treatment. These data suggest, that PEEL is a treatment option in patients with late-stage EPS that can be performed with acceptable morbidity (unpublished data).

Over a study period of two to 19 years, reported mortality rates vary from 25.5 to 56.6% especially in the first year after diagnosis (table 2). In our study including only late-stage EPS patients, three patients (10%) died within the first year after operative treatment, which is a favourable mortality rate (unpubslihed data). The overall mortality rate in our study with 42 EPS patients (31 of them required major surgery due to bowel obstruction) was 21.4%. To achieve such good outcome data, we believe, that these patients should be treated in specialized referral centers.

6. Conclusion

EPS is a rare complication of PD. There are three diagnostic pillars in EPS. clinical, radiological and histologic criteria. However a standardized approach is still lacking, histological analysis of peritoneal biopsies is important tool in the diagnosis of EPS. Peritoneal biopsies should be taken from all patients on PD at any time of surgery (e.g. catheter insertion, correction of a catheter malposition, catheter removal or any other abdominal surgery). Immunosuppressive therapy in patients with advanced disease might not be mandatory due to low degree of acute inflammation in these stages and the lack of prospective trials. Remarkably, time of first clinical symptoms consistent with to requirement of major surgery is very short. Therefore earlier diagnosis of the disease is mandatory, even in asymptomatic patients. Optimized operative therapy with PEEL represents a favourable treatment option in late stage EPS patients, which results in a low mortality and an acceptable morbidity rate.

Compared to the mortality rate of an age-matched dialysis population, outcome of patients even with severe EPS is not worse, if these patients are treated in specialized referral centers.

Author details

Joerg Latus[1], Christoph Ulmer[2], Martin Kimmel[1], M. Dominik Alscher[1] and Niko Braun[1*]

*Address all correspondence to: Niko.braun@rbk.de

1 Department of Internal Medicine, Division of Nephrology, Robert-Bosch-Hospital, Stuttgart, Germany

2 Department of General, Visceral and Trauma Surgery, Robert-Bosch-Hospital, Stuttgart, Germany

References

[1] Brown, M. C, Simpson, K, Kerssens, J. J, & Mactier, R. A. Encapsulating peritoneal sclerosis in the new millennium: a national cohort study. Clin J Am Soc Nephrol. (2009). Epub 2009/06/23., 4(7), 1222-9.

[2] Johnson, D. W, Cho, Y, Livingston, B. E, Hawley, C. M, Mcdonald, S. P, Brown, F. G, et al. Encapsulating peritoneal sclerosis: incidence, predictors, and outcomes. Kidney Int. (2010). Epub 2010/04/09., 77(10), 904-12.

[3] Summers, A. M, Clancy, M. J, Syed, F, Harwood, N, Brenchley, P. E, Augustine, T, et al. Single-center experience of encapsulating peritoneal sclerosis in patients on peritoneal dialysis for end-stage renal failure. Kidney Int. (2005). Epub 2005/10/14., 68(5), 2381-8.

[4] Rigby, R. J, & Hawley, C. M. Sclerosing peritonitis: the experience in Australia. Nephrol Dial Transplant. (1998). Epub 1998/03/03., 13(1), 154-9.

[5] Kawanishi, H, Kawaguchi, Y, Fukui, H, Hara, S, Imada, A, Kubo, H, et al. Encapsulating peritoneal sclerosis in Japan: a prospective, controlled, multicenter study. Am J Kidney Dis. (2004). Epub 2004/09/24., 44(4), 729-37.

[6] Kawaguchi, Y, Kawanishi, H, Mujais, S, Topley, N, & Oreopoulos, D. G. Encapsulating peritoneal sclerosis: definition, etiology, diagnosis, and treatment. International Society for Peritoneal Dialysis Ad Hoc Committee on Ultrafiltration Management in Peritoneal Dialysis. Perit Dial Int. (2000). Suppl 4:SEpub 2000/12/01., 43-55.

[7] Summers, A. M, Abrahams, A. C, Alscher, M. D, Betjes, M, Boeschoten, E. W, Braun, N, et al. A collaborative approach to understanding EPS: the European perspective. Perit Dial Int. (2011). Epub 2011/05/11., 31(3), 245-8.

[8] Kawanishi, H, Moriishi, M, & Tsuchiya, S. Experience of 100 surgical cases of encapsulating peritoneal sclerosis: investigation of recurrent cases after surgery. Advances in peritoneal dialysis Conference on Peritoneal Dialysis. (2006). Epub 2006/09/21., 22, 60-4.

[9] Kawanishi, H, Moriishi, M, Ide, K, & Dohi, K. Recommendation of the surgical option for treatment of encapsulating peritoneal sclerosis. Peritoneal dialysis international : journal of the International Society for Peritoneal Dialysis. (2008). Suppl 3:SEpub 2008/09/20., 205-10.

[10] Oules, R, Challah, S, & Brunner, F. P. Case-control study to determine the cause of sclerosing peritoneal disease. Nephrol Dial Transplant. (1988). Epub 1988/01/01., 3(1), 66-9.

[11] Nomoto, Y, Kawaguchi, Y, Kubo, H, Hirano, H, Sakai, S, & Kurokawa, K. Sclerosing encapsulating peritonitis in patients undergoing continuous ambulatory peritoneal

dialysis: a report of the Japanese Sclerosing Encapsulating Peritonitis Study Group. Am J Kidney Dis. (1996). Epub 1996/09/01., 28(3), 420-7.

[12] Fieren, M. W, Betjes, M. G, Korte, M. R, & Boer, W. H. Posttransplant encapsulating peritoneal sclerosis: a worrying new trend? Perit Dial Int. (2007). Epub 2007/11/07., 27(6), 619-24.

[13] Braun, N, Fritz, P, Biegger, D, Kimmel, M, Reimold, F, Ulmer, C, et al. Difference in the expression of hormone receptors and fibrotic markers in the human peritoneum--implications for therapeutic targets to prevent encapsulating peritoneal sclerosis. Perit Dial Int. (2011). Epub 2011/04/02., 31(3), 291-300.

[14] Kawanishi, H, & Moriishi, M. Epidemiology of encapsulating peritoneal sclerosis in Japan. Perit Dial Int. (2005). Suppl 4:SEpub 2005/11/23., 14-8.

[15] Brown, E. A, Van Biesen, W, Finkelstein, F. O, Hurst, H, Johnson, D. W, Kawanishi, H, et al. Length of time on peritoneal dialysis and encapsulating peritoneal sclerosis: position paper for ISPD. Perit Dial Int. (2009). Epub 2009/11/17., 29(6), 595-600.

[16] Nakamoto, H. Encapsulating peritoneal sclerosis--a clinician's approach to diagnosis and medical treatment. Perit Dial Int. (2005). Suppl 4:SEpub 2005/11/23., 30-8.

[17] Latus, J, Ulmer, C, Fritz, P, Rettenmaier, B, Biegger, D, Lang, T, et al. Encapsulating peritoneal sclerosis: a rare, serious but potentially curable complication of peritoneal dialysis-experience of a referral centre in Germany. Nephrol Dial Transplant. (2012).

[18] Lambie, M. L, John, B, Mushahar, L, Huckvale, C, & Davies, S. J. The peritoneal osmotic conductance is low well before the diagnosis of encapsulating peritoneal sclerosis is made. Kidney Int. (2010). Epub 2010/06/24., 78(6), 611-8.

[19] Tarzi, R. M, Lim, A, Moser, S, Ahmad, S, George, A, Balasubramaniam, G, et al. Assessing the validity of an abdominal CT scoring system in the diagnosis of encapsulating peritoneal sclerosis. Clin J Am Soc Nephrol. (2008). Epub 2008/08/01., 3(6), 1702-10.

[20] Ti, J. P, Al-aradi, A, Conlon, P. J, Lee, M. J, & Morrin, M. M. Imaging features of encapsulating peritoneal sclerosis in continuous ambulatory peritoneal dialysis patients. AJR American journal of roentgenology. (2010). WEpub 2010/06/23., 50-4.

[21] Vlijm, A, Stoker, J, Bipat, S, Spijkerboer, A. M, Phoa, S. S, Maes, R, et al. Computed tomographic findings characteristic for encapsulating peritoneal sclerosis: a case-control study. Perit Dial Int. (2009). Epub 2009/09/25., 29(5), 517-22.

[22] Brown, E. A. Computed tomographic scanning and diagnosis of encapsulating peritoneal sclerosis. Perit Dial Int. (2009). Epub 2009/09/25., 29(5), 502-4.

[23] Augustine, T, Brown, P. W, Davies, S. D, Summers, A. M, & Wilkie, M. E. Encapsulating peritoneal sclerosis: clinical significance and implications. Nephron Clin Pract. (2009). cdiscussion c54. Epub 2009/01/17., 149-54.

[24] Braun, N. Encapsulating Peritoneal Sclerosis- An Overview. Nephrol Ther. (2011).

[25] Honda, K, Nitta, K, Horita, S, Tsukada, M, Itabashi, M, Nihei, H, et al. Histologic criteria for diagnosing encapsulating peritoneal sclerosis in continuous ambulatory peritoneal dialysis patients. Advances in peritoneal dialysis Conference on Peritoneal Dialysis. (2003). Epub 2004/02/07., 19, 169-75.

[26] Garosi, G. Di Paolo N, Sacchi G, Gaggiotti E. Sclerosing peritonitis: a nosological entity. Perit Dial Int. (2005). Suppl 3:SEpub 2005/07/29., 110-2.

[27] Sherif, A. M, Yoshida, H, Maruyama, Y, Yamamoto, H, Yokoyama, K, Hosoya, T, et al. Comparison between the pathology of encapsulating sclerosis and simple sclerosis of the peritoneal membrane in chronic peritoneal dialysis. Therapeutic apheresis and dialysis : official peer-reviewed journal of the International Society for Apheresis, the Japanese Society for Apheresis, the Japanese Society for Dialysis Therapy. (2008). Epub 2008/02/09., 12(1), 33-41.

[28] Nakamura, S, & Niwa, T. Advanced glycation end-products and peritoneal sclerosis. Semin Nephrol. (2004). Epub 2004/10/19., 24(5), 502-5.

[29] Schwenger, V, Morath, C, Salava, A, Amann, K, Seregin, Y, Deppisch, R, et al. Damage to the peritoneal membrane by glucose degradation products is mediated by the receptor for advanced glycation end-products. J Am Soc Nephrol. (2006). Epub 2005/12/02., 17(1), 199-207.

[30] Aroeira, L. S, Aguilera, A, Sanchez-tomero, J. A, & Bajo, M. A. del Peso G, Jimenez-Heffernan JA, et al. Epithelial to mesenchymal transition and peritoneal membrane failure in peritoneal dialysis patients: pathologic significance and potential therapeutic interventions. J Am Soc Nephrol. (2007). Epub 2007/06/15., 18(7), 2004-13.

[31] Alscher, D. M, Braun, N, Biegger, D, & Fritz, P. Peritoneal mast cells in peritoneal dialysis patients, particularly in encapsulating peritoneal sclerosis patients. Am J Kidney Dis. (2007). Epub 2007/03/06., 49(3), 452-61.

[32] Honda, K, & Oda, H. Pathology of encapsulating peritoneal sclerosis. Perit Dial Int. (2005). Suppl 4:SEpub 2005/11/23., 19-29.

[33] Schmidt, D. W, & Flessner, M. F. Pathogenesis and treatment of encapsulating peritoneal sclerosis: basic and translational research. Perit Dial Int. (2008). Suppl 5:SEpub 2008/12/17., 10-5.

[34] Kawanishi, H, Harada, Y, Noriyuki, T, Kawai, T, Takahashi, S, Moriishi, M, et al. Treatment options for encapsulating peritoneal sclerosis based on progressive stage. Advances in peritoneal dialysis Conference on Peritoneal Dialysis. (2001). Epub 2001/08/21., 17, 200-4.

[35] Yamamoto, H, Nakayama, M, Yamamoto, R, Otsuka, Y, Takahashi, H, Kato, N, et al. Fifteen cases of encapsulating peritoneal sclerosis related to peritoneal dialysis: a single-center experience in Japan. Adv Perit Dial. (2002). Epub 2002/10/31., 18, 135-8.

[36] Wong, C. F, Beshir, S, Khalil, A, Pai, P, & Ahmad, R. Successful treatment of encapsulating peritoneal sclerosis with azathioprine and prednisolone. Perit Dial Int. (2005). Epub 2005/06/29., 25(3), 285-7.

[37] Bozkurt, D, Cetin, P, Sipahi, S, Hur, E, Nar, H, Ertilav, M, et al. The effects of renin-angiotensin system inhibition on regression of encapsulating peritoneal sclerosis. Perit Dial Int. (2008). Suppl 5:SEpub 2008/12/17., 38-42.

[38] Nakamoto, H, Imai, H, Fukushima, R, Ishida, Y, Yamanouchi, Y, & Suzuki, H. Role of the renin-angiotensin system in the pathogenesis of peritoneal fibrosis. Perit Dial Int. (2008). Suppl 3:SEpub 2008/09/20., 83-7.

[39] Van Bommel, E. F, Hendriksz, T. R, Huiskes, A. W, & Zeegers, A. G. Brief communication: tamoxifen therapy for nonmalignant retroperitoneal fibrosis. Ann Intern Med. (2006). Epub 2006/01/19., 144(2), 101-6.

[40] del Peso GBajo MA, Gil F, Aguilera A, Ros S, Costero O, et al. Clinical experience with tamoxifen in peritoneal fibrosing syndromes. Advances in peritoneal dialysis Conference on Peritoneal Dialysis. (2003). Epub 2004/02/07., 19, 32-5.

[41] Eltoum, M. A, Wright, S, Atchley, J, & Mason, J. C. Four consecutive cases of peritoneal dialysis-related encapsulating peritoneal sclerosis treated successfully with tamoxifen. Perit Dial Int. (2006). Epub 2006/04/21., 26(2), 203-6.

[42] Korte, M. R, Fieren, M. W, Sampimon, D. E, Lingsma, H. F, Weimar, W, & Betjes, M. G. Tamoxifen is associated with lower mortality of encapsulating peritoneal sclerosis: results of the Dutch Multicentre EPS Study. Nephrol Dial Transplant. (2010). Epub 2010/06/30.

[43] Suga, H, Teraoka, S, Ota, K, Komemushi, S, Furutani, S, Yamauchi, S, et al. Preventive effect of pirfenidone against experimental sclerosing peritonitis in rats. Exp Toxicol Pathol. (1995). Epub 1995/09/01., 47(4), 287-91.

[44] incapsulata) WPÜZpcfBrunns Beitr Klin Chir. (1921).

[45] Braun, N, Alscher, M. D, Kimmel, M, Amann, K, & Buttner, M. Encapsulating peritoneal sclerosis- an overview. Nephrol Ther. (2011). Epub 2011/04/05., 7(3), 162-71.

[46] Gandhi, V. C, Humayun, H. M, Ing, T. S, Daugirdas, J. T, Jablokow, V. R, Iwatsuki, S, et al. Sclerotic thickening of the peritoneal membrane in maintenance peritoneal dialysis patients. Archives of internal medicine. (1980). Epub 1980/09/01., 140(9), 1201-3.

[47] Celicout, B, Levard, H, Hay, J, Msika, S, Fingerhut, A, & Pelissier, E. Sclerosing encapsulating peritonitis: early and late results of surgical management in 32 cases. French Associations for Surgical Research. Digestive surgery. (1998). Epub 1998/12/09., 15(6), 697-702.

Section 3

Systemic Complications Associated to Peritoneal Dialysis

Chapter 4

Inflammation in Peritoneal Dialysis

Joseph C.K. Leung, Loretta Y. Y. Chan,
Kar Neng Lai and Sydney C.W. Tang

Additional information is available at the end of the chapter

http://dx.doi.org/10.5772/55964

1. Introduction

The prevalence of kidney disease has grown continuously. The loss of kidney function during acute kidney disease may occur rapidly and reversibly, and most unfortunately, may progress to end-stage renal disease (ESRD) in which renal replacement therapy (RRT) is required. Due to the short supply of donor kidneys, RRT is now dominated by dialysis. Dialysis can be applied intermittently or continuously using extracorporeal (hemodialysis or HD) or para-corporeal (peritoneal dialysis or PD) methods. Among patients with ESRD, the choice of PD or HD varies considerably from country to country and is related to non-medical factors such as finance, physician preferences, and social culture [1]. It has been suggested that PD should be offered as the first-line dialysis modality [2]. Compared with HD, PD offers better preservation of residual renal function, lower risk of infection with hepatitis B and C, better outcome after transplantation, preservation of vascular access, easy to place on home therapy, simplicity of the technique, and lower costs [3, 4]. The predominant problems associated with PD are ultrafiltration failure and peritonitis. Dialysis patients after an episode of peritonitis may still be affected by prolonged systemic chronic inflammation [5]. Likewise, PD maintains a state of intraperitoneal micro-inflammation that affects the structure and function of the peritoneal membrane, and impairs ultrafiltration efficiency. An understanding of the mechanism in peritoneal inflammation will provide new insight to better preserve the function of the peritoneum membrane, with a goal to improve the quality of life in patients under PD.

2. Inflammatory response during peritoneal dialysis

Inflammation is the body's natural defense involving cascades of immediate immunological responses towards various stimuli, including pathogens, necrotic cells, injury, or irritants.

Acute inflammation is a protective machinery by which the injurious stimuli will be removed and the healing process initiated. On the other hand, chronic inflammation develops if the conditions causing acute inflammation is not resolved over a period of time. Intriguingly, chronic inflammation may be due to excessive physiological responses, such as the wound repairing process, which are intrinsically essential for maintaining normal life. Certain stimuli may directly provoke chronic rather than acute inflammation. Peritoneal inflammation of the microenvironment in the peritoneal cavity during PD generally presents in two major forms: (i) acute inflammation triggered by microbial infection, and (ii) low-grade inflammation or "para-inflammation" under various exogenous or endogenous stimulations during PD. These two forms of inflammation affects the membrane structure and function, and is associated with increased mortality.

2.1. Acute inflammation in PD

The most common form of acute inflammation of peritoneum in PD is peritonitis, which is a serious and the most frequent complication leading to hospitalization and catheter loss [6, 7]. Peritonitis causes a high infection-related mortality in PD patients [8, 9]. The leading cause of PD-associated peritonitis is contamination, predominately with the microorganisms from skin and environment, which is most commonly occur during the dialysis procedure such as PD exchange [10]. Exit site infection (ESI) in which transmigration of microorganisms from the exit site along the PD catheter into the peritoneal cavity, may cause tunnel infections and peritonitis [11, 12]. Enteric peritonitis is a less common cause but important, due to the severity of the inflammation process [13]. Fungal peritonitis accounts for about 4–6% of episodes of the total incidence of the peritonitis, and is with high mortality [14]. Rapidly resolving the infection is the primary approach to treat peritonitis, even if this involve the need for prompt removal of the peritoneal catheter. Before the causative microorganism is identified, initial therapy with broad spectrum antibiotic which is active against the most commonly occurring organisms, will be given according to the guideline from the International Society for Peritoneal Dialysis (ISPD) [9]. It is recommended that in addition to the standard initial protocol, specific regime tailored to the geographic and cultural characteristics, the relevant organisms and their antibiotic resistance pattern should be considered [15]. Detailed examination of the causality of infection-related peritonitis is important for the management. The molecular pathways of inflammation induced by different microbial pathogens are somehow redundant, yet also complex and diverse [16, 17].

2.2. Chronic inflammation in PD

An inherent immune dysfunction in PD patients and the continuous non-specific immune cell stimulation by dialysis procedure contribute to the chronic inflammatory state of patients under the long-term dialysis [18]. Patients on maintenance PD have increased intra-peritoneal levels of hyaluronan and cytokines including interleukin (IL)-1β, IL-6 and transforming growth factor-β (TGF-β) [19, 20]. Chronic inflammation remains an important cause of morbidity in patients with ESRD. During continuous ambulatory peritoneal dialysis (CAPD), peritoneal cells are repeatedly exposed to non-physiologic dialysis fluid (PDF) with low pH and high glucose [21]. PDF also contains toxic substance like glucose degradation products (GDP) generated during the sterilization process and the advanced glycation end products (AGE), which can be formed by amadori reaction between sugar and protein during long-term PD [22]. Dialysis patients are likely to gain fat mass following absorption of glucose from the peritoneal dialysate [23]. Adipocyte in adipose tissue is the major source of adipokines such as leptin, adiponectin and other inflammatory mediators. Adipose tissue is also an important contributor to the peritoneal and systemic inflammation [24, 25]. Exposure of peritoneal cells to the non-physiological dialysate during CAPD leads to "para-inflammation" [26], which is a protective mechanism helping the peritoneum to adapt to the noxious conditions during PD and to restore peritoneum functionality. Regrettably, after repeated exposure to various insults in PDF, dysregulated para-inflammation may eventually develop chronically to inflammatory states associated with ultrafiltration failure. A key feature of chronic inflammation is peritoneal fibrosis [27, 28], in which fibroblasts proliferate or are recruited to the inflamed peritoneum with the activation of cascades of inflammatory or fibrotic cytokines [29, 30].

3. The Mechanisms and pathways of inflammation in PD

The inflammatory pathway of PD consists of modulators, mediators and effectors. A simplified schema for PD-related inflammation is illustrated in Figure 1. The complex interaction among the components involved and the related machinery will determine the outcome of the immune response induced by PD.

3.1. Modulators:

Modulators of PD-related inflammation can be exogenous or endogenous. It should be noted that exogenous modulators may promote or amplify the effects of the endogenous modulators during the process of PD-related inflammation. Intriguingly, the interaction between modulators and the ongoing inflammatory events may form a vicious cycle to amplify the inflammatory process.

3.1.1. Exogenous modulators

The innate immune system recognized catheters used for PD as the foreign bodies. Severe biofilm formation on the catheters have been observed in PD patients without detectable infection [31]. Histologic and functional evidences obtained from rodent model have shown that the catheter insertion may have induced a classic inflammatory reaction characterized by formation of fibrin clots in the peritoneum [32]. Mechanical stress during PD is related to the infiltration of large volume of PDF, especially for achieving specific target of small solute clearance. Volume stress during PD are associated with significant increments in endothelin (ET)-1, a vasoactive peptide that may induce peritoneal fibrosis and indirectly contribute to technique failure in CAPD [33]. ET-1 induces the release of proinflammatory cytokines and increases the deposition of extracellular matrix (ECM) by regulating production and turnover of matrix components. In addition, high fill volumes increase circulating norepinephrine levels

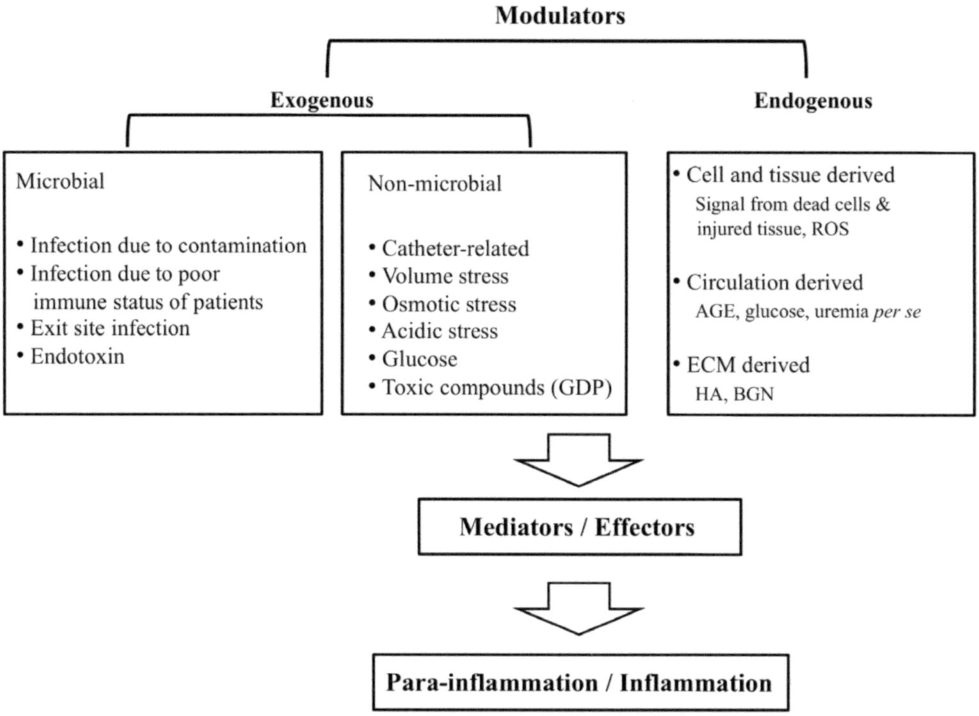

Figure 1. Pathway of the development of PD-related inflammation

[34], blood pressure, intraperitoneal pressure [35], and elicit proinflammatory effects by increasing peritoneal IL-6 and tumor necrosis factor-α (TNF-α) concentration [36]. During PD, cells lining the peritoneal cavity are exposed from time to time to the hyperosmotic environment, and this osmotic stress induces apoptosis of the peritoneal cells [37, 38]. Local acidosis occurs artificially during PD due to the non-physiological properties of PDF which has an acidic pH value. Exposure of macrophages to an acidic environment leads to the increased production of TNF-α through the up-regulation of inducible nitric oxide synthase (iNOS) activity and the activation of nuclear factor-κB (NF-κB) [39]. On the contrary, low pH PDF lead to rapid intracellular acidification and suppression of host defense activity [40, 41]. The acidic PDF induces stress on the endoplasmic reticulum (ER) and suppresses the induction of monocyte chemotactic protein-1 (MCP-1) in the peritoneum through de-activation of NF-κB pathway [42, 43], and this may impair the peritoneal defense mechanisms by interfering with migration of phagocytic cells. Obviously, further study is needed to clarify the role of acidic-stress on PD-related inflammation. High glucose content in PDF induces immunological, structural and functional abnormalities in peritoneal cells during CAPD [44, 45]. High glucose induces vascular inflammatory processes through up-regulation of endothelial cell adhesion molecules, reduction of nitric oxide (NO) release, activation of reactive oxygen species (ROS) and NF-κB [46, 47]. Storage or heat sterilization of PDF generates the toxic substances GDP. Dialysis with GDP-containing PDF is associated with increased vascular endothelial growth

factor (VEGF) production and peritoneal vascularization [48]. GDP decrease the expression of tight junction associated protein, zonula occludens protein 1 (ZO-1), in human peritoneal mesothelial cells (HPMC) *via* the VEGF [49]. Glucose or GDP in PDF may cause AGE formation, which further provoke additional inflammatory stimuli on the peritoneal environment under PD [22, 50, 51]. Contamination and the inherent poor immune status of the PD patients contribute to the microbial stress during PD. Microbial contamination or ESI during PD may evolve to peritonitis, which elicits a virulent acute inflammatory response and is an important cause of hospitalization, catheter loss, and technique failure. The most common contaminated micro-organisms are coagulase-negative *Staphylococcus, S. aureus, Streptococcus*, and Gram-negative bacteria. Much less common are mycobacterium and fungal peritonitis. Skin organisms contamination including *Staphylococcus, Corynebacterium, and Bacillus* species cause mild inflammatory responses. Exit site infection with *Staphylococcus epidermidis* or *Pseudomonas aeruginosa* is difficult to treat, with frequent progression to tunnel infections and peritonitis. Fungal peritonitis generally requires catheter removal. It is worth mentioned that sustained inflammation is observed in patients on PD with peritonitis even after resolution of the clinical symptoms of peritonitis [52]. The C-reactive protein (CRP) remains significantly higher than baseline by day 42 after an episode of peritonitis [5]. Release of neutrophil gelatinase-associated lipocalin (NGAL) into the peritoneal dialysate effluent (PDE) by HPMC is induced following an acute episode of CAPD-related peritonitis, and is related to the up-regulation of the IL-1β concentration [53]. Lipopolysaccharide (LPS), a major component of Gram-negative bacterial cell walls, is a potent immuno-stimulatory product [54]. Endotoxemia is common in PD patients and circulating LPS may derived from the gastrointestinal tract during enteric peritonitis [55]. The level of circulating LPS correlates with the severity of systemic inflammation, suggesting that endotoxemia may contribute to accelerated atherosclerosis in PD patients.

3.1.2. Endogenous modulators

Uremia is associated with the immune dysfunction and is a significant risk factor for cardiovascular abnormalities and death in chronic kidney disease (CKD) patients [56], and this risk is further increased when CKD has progressed to ESRD requiring dialysis. Dialysis decreases the impact of uremia, yet does not remove it completely. In PD patients, uremia fuels the inflammatory state and introduces stress on the peritoneum due to the formation of carbonyl products. It accelerates the formation of advanced oxidation protein products (AOPP) and AGE, that induces an upregulation of the receptors of advanced glycation end products (RAGE) [57]. Binding of AGE to RAGE alone [58], or in combination with the Toll-like receptor (TLR)s, elicits the inflammatory activity [59]. It has been suggested that the high-mobility group box 1 protein (HMGB1) may play a central role in mediating inflammation, and interactions involving the HMGB1-TLR-RAGE axis trigger NF-κB activation and proinflammatory cytokines induction [60]. Cytotoxic injury to mesothelial cells induces ROS, depletes ATP, and triggers the extracellular release of HMGB1, which initiates a chronic inflammatory response [61]. Serum adipokine levels are significantly elevated in uremic patients with CKD [62], and elevated plasma concentrations of adiponectin and leptin have been reported [63, 64]. Leptin activates immune system and serves as a mediator of inflammation [65]. Glucose-based PDF induces a higher leptin secretion by a murine adipocyte cell line 3T3-L1 compared to dialysate with physiological glucose concentration *via* the hexosamine pathway [66]. We have demonstrated that the full-length isoform of leptin receptor, Ob-Rb, is expressed in HPMC and its expression is up-regulated following exposure to glucose [67]. Glucose increases leptin synthesis by peritoneal adipocytes and the adipocyte-derived leptin can induce TGF-β production by HPMC through the Ob-Rb [67]. Adiponectin exerts protective functions on innate and adaptive immunity, including the reduction of phagocytic activity, IL-6 and TNF-α production by macrophage, T-cell response, and the induction of anti-inflammatory cytokines by monocytes, macrophages and dendritic cells [68]. In a recent study using rat PD model, glucose-based PDF down-regulates adiponectin synthesis by adipocytes through an increased ROS generation [69].

In uremic patients under PD, chronic inflammatory processes induce the oxidative stress, generating excess ROS, reactive nitrogen species (RNS), and DNA-reactive aldehydes. These pro-oxidants overwhelm *in vivo* antioxidant defenses, and lead to increased oxidative damage of peritoneal structure and function [70]. The link between oxidative stress and inflammation has been demonstrated in liver injury, where oxidative stress induces the proinflammatory signaling and macrophage activation [71]. In HPMC, ROS amplifies the high glucose-induced expression of fibronectin [72], angiotensin II (AngII) and TGF-β [44].

Heat-shock proteins (HSP), a marker of the cellular stress response, is the main effector of the cellular reparative machinery. Induction of HSP expression will counteract cellular injury caused by PDF exposure. PDF induces HSP release by cultured HPMC [73, 74]. In an experimental model of PD, PDF infusion causes cellular injury but also up-regulates HSP-72 [75]. In HPMC under sublethal injury, secretion of HSP-72 correlates with the release of proinflammatory IL-8 [76].

Breakdown products of the ECM during tissue injury, may serve as the endogenous modulator of inflammation. There is growing evidence that ECM molecules may deliver proinflammatory signals [77, 78]. In the context of PD, expression and release of hyaluronan (HA) and biglycan (BGN) is well recognized. HPMC synthesize and secrete ECM proteins including BGN and HA, which are detectable in PDE [19, 79, 80]. Under physiological conditions, HA is present as an inert high-molecular-weight polymer. Upon tissue injury, HA is broken down into inflammatory low-molecular-weight fragments, which activate the TLR4 and promote either an inflammatory or a tissue-repair response [81, 82]. Other than HA, BGN also implicate in modulating the proinflammatory functions. BGN can act as a "danger" motif, a potential innate antigen analogous to pathogen-associated molecular pattern (PAMP), which signal through TLR4 and TLR2 to initiate the inflammatory cascade [83]. BGN binds with TGF-β and TNF-α to regulate the proinflammatory cytokine activity [84, 85]. Markedly elevated TNF-α and IL-1β is found in PDE from CAPD patients with peritonitis [86]. The activity of proinflammatory master cytokine IL-1β is regulated by sequentially synthesis and cleavage of pro-IL-1 by caspase-1 (also named as IL-1 converting enzyme) [87, 88]. The production of pro-IL-1 is signaled by TLR and the activation of caspase-1 requires the assembly and activity of a cytosolic multi-protein complex known as the inflammasome, consisting of nucleotide-binding oligomerization-like receptor family members (NLRs) [89]. NLRP3 is the best characterized NLRs which recruits caspase-1 to the inflammasome. In macrophage, soluble BGN induces the NLRP3 inflammasome, activating caspase-1 and releasing mature IL-1β [90]. Most notably, the pro-inflammatory events initiated by HA or BGN are also ROS dependent [91]. Figure 2 illustrates the complex interaction amount various endogenous modulators in relation to peritoneal inflammation.

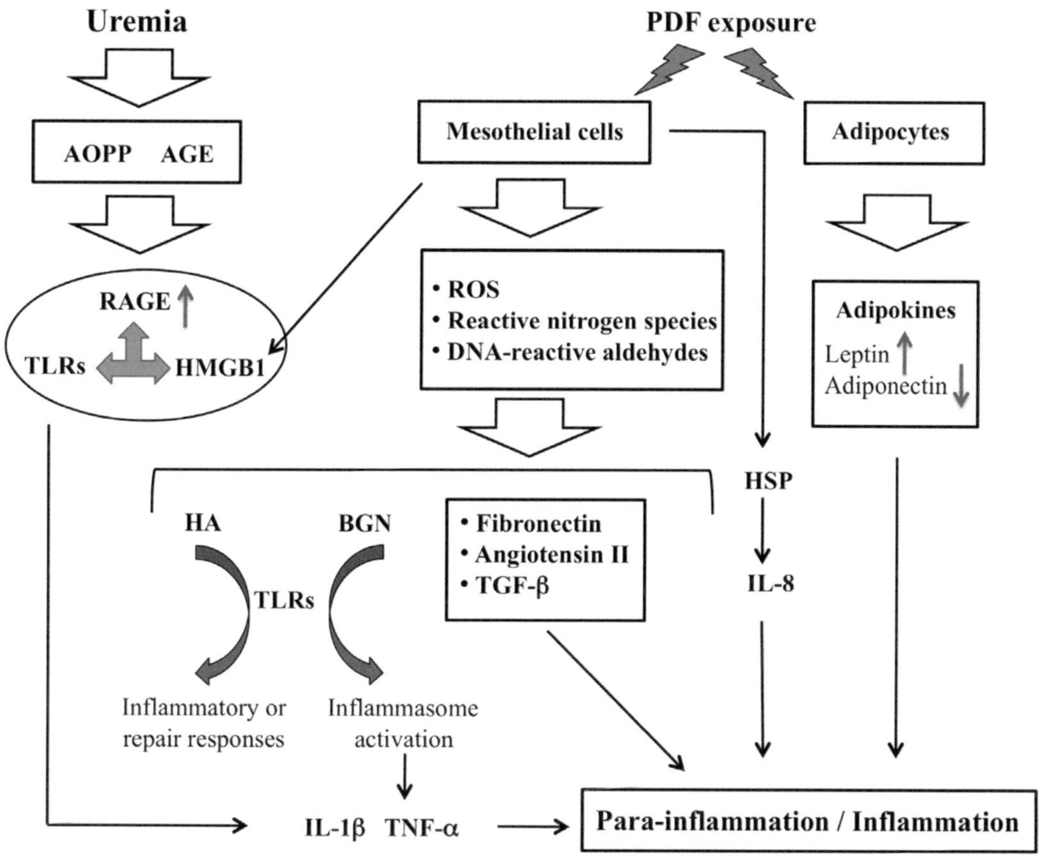

Figure 2. Endogenous modulators in the regulation of peritoneal inflammation

4. Mediators

An array of inflammatory mediators is significantly induced or up-regulated following PD, and is known to modulate the structure and function of the peritoneal membrane, as well as the function of the downstream effectors of the inflammatory pathway. Of equally important, these mediators also play a central role in the maintenance of homeostasis in peritoneum. These mediators are either derived from plasma proteins or secreted by infiltrating or resident peritoneal cells. While many of these inflammatory mediators have overlapped effects on the vasculature and on the recruitment of leukocytes, other mediators may perform additional specific functions and are produced directly in response to particular stimulation by PD-related modulators. It should be noted that some mediators can induce the production of other inflammatory mediators and it is important to understand the logic underlying this hierarchy of mediators induction. The soluble mediators of PD-related inflammation classified according to their biochemical properties is shown in Table 1.

Acute Phase Proteins		**Chemokines and Circulating Adhesion Molecules**		
CRP		IL-8	sICAM-1	
NGAL		MIF	sVCAM-1	
		MCP-1	RANTES	
		SDF-1		
Complement Components		**Cytokines and Adipokines**		
C3	C3a	CTGF	TNF-α	Adiponectin
C4	C4a	IFN-γ	TGF-β	Apelin
C5a	Crry	IL-1	VEGF	Leptin
CD59		IL-6	RBP-4	HGF
		FGF-2		
Lipid Mediators		**Vasoactive Substances**		
PGE2		Histamine	PRA	
PAF		AngII	ET	
5-LOX		ANP		
Proteolytic Enzymes				
MMP-2, 3, 7, 9				
TIMP-1				
Tryptase				

There are many other members in each category, only those commonly reported are listed.

Table 1. Mediators of PD-related inflammation

4.1. Acute phase proteins

Emerging evidences have suggested that acute phase proteins generated during PD may have additional function instead of just serving as the markers of inflammation. CRP plays a proinflammatory role in activating monocyte chemotactic protein [92]. Data from studies on endothelial cells, monocytes-macrophages and smooth muscle cells support a direct role for CRP in atherogenesis [93-95]. NGAL has been evaluated as an urinary biomarker for detecting the early onset of renal tubular cell injury [96]. In CAPD, NGAL in PDE is a marker for neutrophil-dependent bacterial peritonitis, and is also synthesized by HPMC induced specifically by IL1-β [53]. NGAL directly involves in the pathogenesis of CKD and cardiovascular abnormality [97].

Residential Effectors:	**Major Soluble Factors**
Adipocyte	Adiponectin, IL-6, leptin, RBP-4
Endothelial cell	MCP-1, IL-6, IL-8, sICAM-1, sVCAM-1
Fibroblast	Collagen, PGE-2, HA, IL-8
Macrophage	PGE2, IL-1, IL-6, IL-8, MCP-1, TNF-α
Mast cell	Histamine, IL-8, TNF-α, TGF-β, tryptase, VEGF
Mesothelial cell	Chemokines, HA, FGF-2, HA, TGF-β, TNF-α,VEGF
Recruited Effectors:	
Lymphocyte	TGF-β, IFN-γ
Macrophage	PGE-2, IL-1, MCP-1, TNF-α
Mast cell	Histamine, tryptase, VEGF
Polymorphonuclear cell	Soluble IL-6, TNF-α, elastase

Table 2. Effectors in PD-related Inflammation

4.2. Chemokines and circulating adhesion molecules

In response to modulators of peritoneal inflammation, chemokines are produced by peritoneal cells including HPMC [98], macrophages [43], adipocytes [99], to control leukocyte extravasation and chemotaxis towards the affected tissues. These chemokines includes IL-8 [98, 100], MCP-1 [98, 101], macrophage inhibitory factor (MIF) [102], and regulated upon activation normal T cell expressed and secreted (RANTES) [98, 101]. Strikingly, HPMC express the α-chemokine stromal derived factor-1 (SDF-1) [103]. The expression levels of SDF-1 is up-regulated by TGF-β1 treatment, resulting in an increased migratory potential of HPMC, which is suggested to be involved in the re-epithelialization of denuded basement membrane at the site of peritoneal injury [104]. Soluble adhesion molecules including soluble intercellular adhesion molecule-1 (sICAM-1) [105] and soluble vascular cell adhesion molecule-1 (sVCAM-1) [106] are produced by endothelial cells during PD, and their concentration correlates with atherogenesis or cardiovascular functions.

4.3. Complement components

Complement activation during PD plays key roles in the maintenance of host homeostasis by eliminating infectious microorganisms and injured cells. Complement activation releases a number of biologically active products that drive peritoneal inflammation [107]. The complement fragments, C3a, C4a and C5a (also known as anaphylatoxins), are produced by several pathways of complement activation. These complement components promote the recruitment of granulocytes and monocytes, and induce mast-cell degranulation, thereby affecting the vasculature of the peritoneum in PD. The synthesis of C3 and C4 by HPMC are regulated by PDF [108]. In rodent model, blocking C5a reduces influx of neutrophils and improve ultrafiltration [109]. Inhibiting the complement activation by complement regulators (CRegs), Crry and CD59, may protect the peritoneal membrane from long-term PD injury [110].

4.4. Cytokines and adipokines

Numerous cytokines are produced by peritoneal cells, infiltrating macrophages or mast cells (Table 1). These cytokines play pluripotent pleiotropic roles in the peritoneal inflammation, participate in the host defense mechanisms and the induction of the acute-phase response. During peritonitis, there is increased release of IL-1β, IL-6, TGF-β and TNF-α by HPMC [52]. These cytokines may autocrinally induce epithelial to mesenchymal transition (EMT) in HPMC, and this further promotes peritoneal inflammation and fibrosis [29, 111, 112]. In the uremic pre-dialysis and PD patients, there is increased peritoneal expression of the fibroblast growth factor-2 (FGF-2) and VEGF [113]. Compared to patients dialysed with low-GDP containing PDF, patients dialysed with less-biocompatible PDF have increased concentration of TNF-α, hepatocyte growth factor (HGF), and IL-6 in the dialysate [102]. AGE and GDP in PDF differentially regulate the synthesis of connective tissue growth factor (CTGF) by peritoneal resident cells. The CTGF synthesis by HPMC can be further amplified by TGF-β released from peritoneal fibroblast or endothelial cells [114]. Crosstalk among peritoneal cells and their cytokines may amply the inflammatory cascade. The differential activation of different transcriptional factors and the diverse response of HPMC towards CTGF, TGF-β and VEGF, suggest that peritoneal cytokines have an overlapping and yet distinct role on peritoneal target cells. Other than the cytokines, peritoneal adipocytes can mediate various physiological processes through the secretion of an array of adipokines including leptin, adiponectin, apelin, retinol-binding protein-4 (RBP-4) [103, 115]. These adipokines have distinct functions on peritoneum during PD. For example, leptin augments myofibroblastic conversion of HPMC [116]. The relative levels of leptin and adiponectin in dialysate from PD patients may indicate the risk of cardiovascular disease [117].

4.5. Lipid mediators

Two major classes of lipid mediators, eicosanoids and platelet-activating factors (PAF), are derived from phosphatidylcholine, a member of the phospholipid family that is present in the inner leaflet of cellular membranes. Prostaglandins E2 (PGE2) is generated from eicosanoids, whereas PAF is produced by the acetylation of lysophosphatidic acid. PGE2 causes vasodilation and modulates the change of peritoneal permeability in PD after peritonitis [118]. PAF activates several processes that occur during the inflammatory response, including the recruitment of leukocytes, vascular permeability and platelet activation. Oxidative stress during PD causes unrestrained synthesis of PAF through interfering the proper function of alpha 1-proteinase inhibitor, a PAF inhibitor, [119]. Esterified eicosanoids are produced from 5-Lipoxygenase (5-LOX) by neutrophils after peritonitis, and enhance the generation of IL-8 and superoxide [120].

4.6. Proteolytic enzymes

Proteolytic enzymes have diverse roles in inflammation, in part through degrading ECM and basement-membrane proteins. These proteases have important roles in many processes, including host defense, tissue remodeling and leukocyte migration. Matrix metalloproteinase (MMP) is the most important family of proteolytic enzymes in mesothelial homeostasis and wound repair. Of equal important is the endogenous tissue inhibitors of metalloproteinase (TIMP), which moderate MMP activity. The balance between MMPs and TIMPs, helps to regulate ECM turnover during tissue remodeling in PD. MMP-2 has been associated with the oxidative stress marker in PD [121]. Activation of MMP-2 causes peritoneal injury during peritoneal dialysis in rats [122]. Neutral-pH PDF improves peritoneal function and decreases MMP-2 in patients undergoing CAPD [123]. MMP-2 and TIMP-1 levels in peritoneal effluents reflect solute transport rate and are associated with peritoneal injury [124]. Regression analysis revealed that both the MMP-7 and TIMP-1, are excellent predictors of cellular stress in dialyzed patients using HSP-27 as the marker [125]. The number of mast cells is increased in PD patients [126], and mast cell tryptase is a serine protease implicated in promoting angiogenesis and fibrosis [126, 127].

4.7. Vasoactive substances

Vasoactive amines modulate the vascular permeability, vasodilation, or vasoconstriction of the peritoneal vasculature during PD, and are produced in an all-or-none manner during degranulation from mast cells and platelets. PDF induces peritoneal histamine release from mast cells [128], and this further causes calcium flux, which activates HPMC and influences cytoskeleton organization [129]. The neuropeptide substance P exaggerates the affected microvascular tone, albumin loss and reduced ultrafiltration in a rat PD model [128]. Plasma levels of atrial natriuretic peptide (ANP), pro-renin activity (PRA), and ET are increased in uremic patients on long-term CAPD, and suggesting the risk of development of myocardial function [130]. AngII activates macrophages and fibroblast to secrete proinflammatory cytokines, chemokines, and VEGF [131]. AngII plays important roles in regulating peritoneal extracellular volume and in the development of peritoneal fibrosis [132, 133].

5. Effectors

The effectors of PD inflammatory response are the residential peritoneal cells and the recruited leukocytes. Residential peritoneal effector cells are adipocytes, endothelial cells, fibroblasts, macrophages, mast cells and mesothelial cells. Recruited leukocytes include polymorphonuclear cells (PMN), T or B lymphocytes, macrophages and mast cells. Table 2 shows the cell types and their released mediators, which are of relevance to the PD-induced inflammation.

Upon PD, both the exogenous or endogenous modulators activate peritoneal adipocytes, macrophages and mesothelial cells, which produce inflammatory cytokines, adipokines and growth factors. These mediators will further promote the secretion of angiogenic factors, fibrotic cytokines and growth factors, by fibroblasts, endothelial cells and mast cells through paracrine interaction. In the meantime, residential HPMC, adipocyte and macrophage also release chemotatic mediators to recruit the exogenous inflammatory immune effectors. All these events orchestrate to amplify the inflammatory cascades and eventually lead to the loss of ultrafiltration and development of peritoneal fibrosis.

6. New PDF and immune responses

Emerging evidences suggest the beneficial effects on peritoneal function by using new PDF with decreasing acidity, reducing GDP concentration, and with non-glucose osmotic agents such as amino acids or glucose polymers. *In vitro* cell culture studies have demonstrated enhanced biocompatibility with improved survival of peritoneal cells exposed to new PDF [134-136]. Data from animal models of PD using new PDF also have shown reduced fibrosis and neoangiogenesis, improved macrophage function, and better maintained ultrafiltration [137, 138]. In humans, the use of glucose-polymer-based solution reduced the cholesterol levels with enhanced lipid oxidation and improved serum profiles of adipokines [139-141]. Despite these beneficial effects, use of glucose-polymer-based solution may increase levels of AGE and other immune mediators including IL-6, TNF-α and HA [142-144]. The use of amino-acid-based PDE improves protein malnutrition but exerts negative metabolic effects of increasing serum urea and homocysteine levels [145]. Moreover, PDE level of IL-6 is increased, reflecting the activation of inflammatory response of the peritoneal membrane [146]. The use of glucose-based neutral pH PDF achieves less activation of peritoneal membrane the best preservation of its integrity. The levels of AGE, HA, VEGF and IL-6 are not altered and the effluent-derived macrophage phagocytic function is enhanced [147-150].

7. Conclusion

The PD-related inflammation is an exceedingly complex process. Although some of the destructive events of PD-induced inflammation can be prevented, nevertheless, other long-term damage is understandably unavoidable. The incidences of peritonitis, exit site infection and catheter malfunction may be decreased with better patient education, optimal exit site care, the use of oral prophylactic antibiotics after wet contamination, and the use of the disconnect systems. The inflammatory modulators in the conventional PDF may be reduced or removed by using novel PDF-based replacement of glucose with icodextrin and amino acids, lactate with bicarbonate at a neutral to physiological pH.

There are potential therapeutic options to minimize peritoneal inflammation in PD patients, but yet need extensive research for further confirmation [151]. Acute peritonitis may be prevented by the use of chemokine receptor blockers, mast cell stabilizers or corticosteroid to block excessive macrophage activity. Chronic PD-related inflammation may be targeted by inhibiting various signaling pathways involved in the inflammatory cascade, or by the introduction of anti-inflammatory agents including anti-RAGE antibodies, bone morphogenetic protein-7 (BMP-7) or Smad7 transgene delivery.

Desperately, if patients have not been given kidney transplant, peritoneum fibrosis will be developed eventually with long term PD. Even after kidney transplant, the restoration and repair of the already injured and thickened peritoneum are still required. Thus, the uppermost challenge is to preserve and at the best, to restore the peritoneum function. Stem cells transplantation either from bone marrow or using mesenchymal stem cells, although still in its infancy, may be an attractive intervention for the repair or replenishment of the cellular reservoir of multi-potential cells of the damaged peritoneal tissue. Further investigation along this direction is warranted.

List of abbreviations

AGE Advanced glycation end products

Ang II Angiotensin II

ANP Atrial natriuretic peptide

AOPP Advanced oxidation protein products

BGN Biglycan

BMP-7 Bone Morphogenetic Protein-7

CAPD Continuous ambulatory peritoneal dialysis

CKD Chronic kidney disease

CRegs Complement regulators

CRP C-reactive protein

GDP Glucose degradation products

ECM Extracellular matrix

EMT Epithelial to mesenchymal transition

ER Endoplasmic reticulum

ESI Exit site infection

ESRD End-stage renal disease

ET Endothelin

FGF-2 Fibroblast growth factor-2

HA Hyaluronan

HD Hemodialysis

HGF Hepatocyte growth factor

HMGB1High-mobility group box 1 protein

HPMC Human peritoneal mesothelial cells

HSP Heat-shock proteins

iNOS Inducible nitric oxide synthase

IFN-γ Interferon- γ

IL Interleukin

ISPD International Society for Peritoneal Dialysis

5-LOX 5-Lipoxygenase

LPS Lipopolysaccharide

MCP-1 Monocyte chemotactic protein-1

MMP Metalloproteinase

NF-κB Nuclear factor-κB

NGAL Neutrophil gelatinase-associated lipocalin

NLRs Nucleotide-binding oligomerization-like receptor family members

PAF Platelet-activating factors

PAMP Pathogen-associated molecular patterns

PD Peritoneal dialysis

PDE Peritoneal dialysate effluent

PGE2 Prostaglandins E2

PDF Peritoneal dialysis fluid

PMN Polymorphonuclear cells

PRA Pro-renin activity

http://dx.doi.org/10.5772/55964

RAGE Receptors of advanced glycation end products

RANTES Regulated upon activation normal T cell expressed and secreted

RBP-4 Retinol-binding protein-4

RNS Reactive nitrogen species

ROS Reactive oxygen species

RRF Renal replacement therapy

SDF-1 Stromal derived factor-1

sICAM-1 Soluble intercellular adhesion molecule-1

sVCAM-1 Soluble vascular cell adhesion molecule-1

TGF-β Transforming growth factor-β

TIMP Tissue inhibitors of metalloproteinases

TLR Toll-like receptor

TNF-α Tumor necrosis factor-α

VEGF Vascular endothelial growth factor

ZO-1 Zonula occludens protein-1

Acknowledgements

We apologize to the investigators whose work was not cited due to space limitations. The study was supported by the Baxter Extramural Grant and was partly supported by L & T Charitable Foundation and the House of INDOCAFE.

Author details

Joseph C.K. Leung[1], Loretta Y. Y. Chan[1], Kar Neng Lai[2] and Sydney C.W. Tang[1]

*Address all correspondence to: jckleung@hku.hk

1 Department of Medicine, Queen Mary Hospital, University of Hong Kong, Pokfulam, Hong Kong, China

2 Nephrology Center, Hong Kong Sanatorium and Hospital, Happy Valley, Hong Kong, China

References

[1] Nissenson AR, Prichard SS, Cheng IK, Gokal R, Kubota M, Maiorca R, Riella MC, Rottembourg J, Stewart JH. ESRD modality selection into the 21st century: the importance of non medical factors. ASAIO J 1997;43(3):143-50.

[2] Chaudhary K, Sangha H, Khanna R. Peritoneal dialysis first: rationale. Clin J Am Soc Nephrol 2011;6(2):447-56.

[3] Berger A, Edelsberg J, Inglese GW, Bhattacharyya SK, Oster G. Cost comparison of peritoneal dialysis versus hemodialysis in end-stage renal disease. Am J Manag Care 2009;15(8):509-18.

[4] Gokal R, Blake PG, Passlick-Deetjen J, Schaub TP, Prichard S, Burkart JM. What is the evidence that peritoneal dialysis is underutilized as an ESRD therapy? Semin Dial 2002;15(3):149-61.

[5] Lam MF, Leung JC, Lo WK, Tam S, Chong MC, Lui SL, Tse KC, Chan TM, Lai KN. Hyperleptinaemia and chronic inflammation after peritonitis predicts poor nutritional status and mortality in patients on peritoneal dialysis. Nephrol Dial Transplant 2007;22(5):1445-50.

[6] Piraino B. Insights on peritoneal dialysis-related infections. Contrib Nephrol 2009;163:161-8.

[7] Fried LF, Bernardini J, Johnston JR, Piraino B. Peritonitis influences mortality in peritoneal dialysis patients. J Am Soc Nephrol 1996;7(10):2176-82.

[8] Perez Fontan M, Rodriguez-Carmona A, Garcia-Naveiro R, Rosales M, Villaverde P, Valdes F. Peritonitis-related mortality in patients undergoing chronic peritoneal dialysis. Perit Dial Int 2005;25(3):274-84.

[9] Li PK, Szeto CC, Piraino B, Bernardini J, Figueiredo AE, Gupta A, Johnson DW, Kuijper EJ, Lye WC, Salzer W, Schaefer F, Struijk DG. Peritoneal dialysis-related infections recommendations: 2010 update. Perit Dial Int 2010;30(4):393-423.

[10] Yap DY, Chu WL, Ng F, Yip TP, Lui SL, Lo WK. Risk Factors and Outcome of Contamination in Patients on Peritoneal Dialysis--a Single-Center Experience of 15 Years. Perit Dial Int 2012.

[11] van Diepen AT, Tomlinson GA, Jassal SV. The Association between Exit Site Infection and Subsequent Peritonitis among Peritoneal Dialysis Patients. Clin J Am Soc Nephrol 2012.

[12] Pecoits-Filho R, Stenvinkel P, Wang AY, Heimburger O, Lindholm B. Chronic inflammation in peritoneal dialysis: the search for the holy grail? Perit Dial Int 2004;24(4):327-39.

[13] Kern EO, Newman LN, Cacho CP, Schulak JA, Weiss MF. Abdominal catastrophe revisited: the risk and outcome of enteric peritoneal contamination. Perit Dial Int 2002;22(3):323-34.

[14] Levallois J, Nadeau-Fredette AC, Labbe AC, Laverdiere M, Ouimet D, Vallee M. Ten-year experience with fungal peritonitis in peritoneal dialysis patients: antifungal susceptibility patterns in a North-American center. Int J Infect Dis 2012;16(1):e41-3.

[15] Li PK, Chow KM. Infectious complications in dialysis--epidemiology and outcomes. Nat Rev Nephrol 2012;8(2):77-88.

[16] Cinel I, Opal SM. Molecular biology of inflammation and sepsis: a primer. Crit Care Med 2009;37(1):291-304.

[17] Feezor RJ, Oberholzer C, Baker HV, Novick D, Rubinstein M, Moldawer LL, Pribble J, Souza S, Dinarello CA, Ertel W, Oberholzer A. Molecular characterization of the acute inflammatory response to infections with gram-negative versus gram-positive bacteria. Infect Immun 2003;71(10):5803-13.

[18] Amore A, Coppo R. Immunological basis of inflammation in dialysis. Nephrol Dial Transplant 2002;17 Suppl 8:16-24.

[19] Lai KN, Szeto CC, Lai KB, Lam CW, Chan DT, Leung JC. Increased production of hyaluronan by peritoneal cells and its significance in patients on CAPD. Am J Kidney Dis 1999;33(2):318-24.

[20] Lai KN, Lai KB, Szeto CC, Lam CW, Leung JC. Growth factors in continuous ambulatory peritoneal dialysis effluent. Their relation with peritoneal transport of small solutes. Am J Nephrol 1999;19(3):416-22.

[21] Di Paolo N, Sacchi G, De Mia M, Gaggiotti E, Capotondo L, Rossi P, Bernini M, Pucci AM, Ibba L, Sabatelli P, et al. Morphology of the peritoneal membrane during continuous ambulatory peritoneal dialysis. Nephron 1986;44(3):204-11.

[22] Lamb EJ, Cattell WR, Dawnay AB. In vitro formation of advanced glycation end products in peritoneal dialysis fluid. Kidney Int 1995;47(6):1768-74.

[23] Axelsson J, Rashid Qureshi A, Suliman ME, Honda H, Pecoits-Filho R, Heimburger O, Lindholm B, Cederholm T, Stenvinkel P. Truncal fat mass as a contributor to inflammation in end-stage renal disease. Am J Clin Nutr 2004;80(5):1222-9.

[24] Axelsson J, Heimburger O, Stenvinkel P. Adipose tissue and inflammation in chronic kidney disease. Contrib Nephrol 2006;151:165-74.

[25] Axelsson J, Heimburger O, Lindholm B, Stenvinkel P. Adipose tissue and its relation to inflammation: the role of adipokines. J Ren Nutr 2005;15(1):131-6.

[26] Medzhitov R. Origin and physiological roles of inflammation. Nature 2008;454(7203): 428-35.

[27] Kaneko K, Hamada C, Tomino Y. Peritoneal fibrosis intervention. Perit Dial Int 2007;27 Suppl 2:S82-6.

[28] Williams JD, Craig KJ, Topley N, Von Ruhland C, Fallon M, Newman GR, Mackenzie RK, Williams GT. Morphologic changes in the peritoneal membrane of patients with renal disease. J Am Soc Nephrol 2002;13(2):470-9.

[29] Margetts PJ, Bonniaud P. Basic mechanisms and clinical implications of peritoneal fibrosis. Perit Dial Int 2003;23(6):530-41.

[30] Lai KN, Tang SC, Leung JC. Mediators of inflammation and fibrosis. Perit Dial Int 2007;27 Suppl 2:S65-71.

[31] Swartz R, Messana J, Holmes C, Williams J. Biofilm formation on peritoneal catheters does not require the presence of infection. ASAIO Trans 1991;37(4):626-34.

[32] Flessner MF. Inflammation from sterile dialysis solutions and the longevity of the peritoneal barrier. Clin Nephrol 2007;68(6):341-8.

[33] Morgera S, Kuchinke S, Budde K, Lun A, Hocher B, Neumayer HH. Volume stress-induced peritoneal endothelin-1 release in continuous ambulatory peritoneal dialysis. J Am Soc Nephrol 1999;10(12):2585-90.

[34] Vlachojannis JG, Tsakas S, Alexandri S, Petropoulou C, Goumenos DS. Continuous ambulatory peritoneal dialysis is responsible for an increase in plasma norepinephrine. Perit Dial Int 2000;20(3):322-7.

[35] de Jesus Ventura M, Amato D, Correa-Rotter R, Paniagua R. Relationship between fill volume, intraperitoneal pressure, body size, and subjective discomfort perception in CAPD patients. Mexican Nephrology Collaborative Study Group. Perit Dial Int 2000;20(2):188-93.

[36] Paniagua R, Ventura Mde J, Rodriguez E, Sil J, Galindo T, Hurtado ME, Alcantara G, Chimalpopoca A, Gonzalez I, Sanjurjo A, Barron L, Amato D, Mujais S. Impact of fill volume on peritoneal clearances and cytokine appearance in peritoneal dialysis. Perit Dial Int 2004;24(2):156-62.

[37] Gastaldello K, Husson C, Dondeyne JP, Vanherweghem JL, Tielemans C. Cytotoxicity of mononuclear cells as induced by peritoneal dialysis fluids: insight into mechanisms that regulate osmotic stress-related apoptosis. Perit Dial Int 2008;28(6):655-66.

[38] Gotloib L. Mechanisms of cell death during peritoneal dialysis. A role for osmotic and oxidative stress. Contrib Nephrol 2009;163:35-44.

[39] Bellocq A, Suberville S, Philippe C, Bertrand F, Perez J, Fouqueray B, Cherqui G, Baud L. Low environmental pH is responsible for the induction of nitric-oxide synthase in macrophages. Evidence for involvement of nuclear factor-kappaB activation. J Biol Chem 1998;273(9):5086-92.

[40] Witowski J, Topley N, Jorres A, Liberek T, Coles GA, Williams JD. Effect of lactate-buffered peritoneal dialysis fluids on human peritoneal mesothelial cell interleukin-6 and prostaglandin synthesis. Kidney Int 1995;47(1):282-93.

[41] Mortier S, Lameire NH, De Vriese AS. The effects of peritoneal dialysis solutions on peritoneal host defense. Perit Dial Int 2004;24(2):123-38.

[42] Johno H, Ogata R, Nakajima S, Hiramatsu N, Kobayashi T, Hara H, Kitamura M. Acidic stress-ER stress axis for blunted activation of NF-kappaB in mesothelial cells exposed to peritoneal dialysis fluid. Nephrol Dial Transplant 2012.

[43] Ogata R, Hiramatsu N, Hayakawa K, Nakajima S, Yao J, Kobayashi T, Kitamura M. Impairment of MCP-1 expression in mesothelial cells exposed to peritoneal dialysis fluid by osmotic stress and acidic stress. Perit Dial Int 2011;31(1):80-9.

[44] Noh H, Ha H, Yu MR, Kim YO, Kim JH, Lee HB. Angiotensin II mediates high glucose-induced TGF-beta1 and fibronectin upregulation in HPMC through reactive oxygen species. Perit Dial Int 2005;25(1):38-47.

[45] Ha H, Yu MR, Lee HB. High glucose-induced PKC activation mediates TGF-beta 1 and fibronectin synthesis by peritoneal mesothelial cells. Kidney Int 2001;59(2): 463-70.

[46] Lee YJ, Kang DG, Kim JS, Lee HS. Effect of Buddleja officinalis on high-glucose-induced vascular inflammation in human umbilical vein endothelial cells. Exp Biol Med (Maywood) 2008;233(6):694-700.

[47] Booth G, Stalker TJ, Lefer AM, Scalia R. Elevated ambient glucose induces acute inflammatory events in the microvasculature: effects of insulin. Am J Physiol Endocrinol Metab 2001;280(6):E848-56.

[48] Park SH, Lee EG, Kim IS, Kim YJ, Cho DK, Kim YL. Effect of glucose degradation products on the peritoneal membrane in a chronic inflammatory infusion model of peritoneal dialysis in the rat. Perit Dial Int 2004;24(2):115-22.

[49] Leung JC, Chan LY, Li FF, Tang SC, Chan KW, Chan TM, Lam MF, Wieslander A, Lai KN. Glucose degradation products downregulate ZO-1 expression in human peritoneal mesothelial cells: the role of VEGF. Nephrol Dial Transplant 2005;20(7): 1336-49.

[50] Tauer A, Zhang X, Schaub TP, Zimmeck T, Niwa T, Passlick-Deetjen J, Pischetsrieder M. Formation of advanced glycation end products during CAPD. Am J Kidney Dis 2003;41(3 Suppl 1):S57-60.

[51] Schwedler S, Schinzel R, Vaith P, Wanner C. Inflammation and advanced glycation end products in uremia: simple coexistence, potentiation or causal relationship? Kidney Int Suppl 2001;78:S32-6.

[52] Lai KN, Lai KB, Lam CW, Chan TM, Li FK, Leung JC. Changes of cytokine profiles during peritonitis in patients on continuous ambulatory peritoneal dialysis. Am J Kidney Dis 2000;35(4):644-52.

[53] Leung JC, Lam MF, Tang SC, Chan LY, Tam KY, Yip TP, Lai KN. Roles of neutrophil gelatinase-associated lipocalin in continuous ambulatory peritoneal dialysis-related peritonitis. J Clin Immunol 2009;29(3):365-78.

[54] Hemmi H, Takeuchi O, Kawai T, Kaisho T, Sato S, Sanjo H, Matsumoto M, Hoshino K, Wagner H, Takeda K, Akira S. A Toll-like receptor recognizes bacterial DNA. Nature 2000;408(6813):740-5.

[55] Szeto CC, Kwan BC, Chow KM, Lai KB, Chung KY, Leung CB, Li PK. Endotoxemia is related to systemic inflammation and atherosclerosis in peritoneal dialysis patients. Clin J Am Soc Nephrol 2008;3(2):431-6.

[56] Wanner C, Zimmermann J, Schwedler S, Metzger T. Inflammation and cardiovascular risk in dialysis patients. Kidney Int Suppl 2002(80):99-102.

[57] De Vriese AS. The John F. Maher Recipient Lecture 2004: Rage in the peritoneum. Perit Dial Int 2005;25(1):8-11.

[58] Hofmann MA, Drury S, Fu C, Qu W, Taguchi A, Lu Y, Avila C, Kambham N, Bierhaus A, Nawroth P, Neurath MF, Slattery T, Beach D, McClary J, Nagashima M, Morser J, Stern D, Schmidt AM. RAGE mediates a novel proinflammatory axis: a central cell surface receptor for S100/calgranulin polypeptides. Cell 1999;97(7):889-901.

[59] Veloso CA, Fernandes JS, Volpe CM, Fagundes-Netto FS, Reis JS, Chaves MM, Nogueira-Machado JA. TLR4 and RAGE: similar routes leading to inflammation in type 2 diabetic patients. Diabetes Metab 2011;37(4):336-42.

[60] Nogueira-Machado JA, Volpe CM, Veloso CA, Chaves MM. HMGB1, TLR and RAGE: a functional tripod that leads to diabetic inflammation. Expert Opin Ther Targets 2011;15(8):1023-35.

[61] Yang H, Rivera Z, Jube S, Nasu M, Bertino P, Goparaju C, Franzoso G, Lotze MT, Krausz T, Pass HI, Bianchi ME, Carbone M. Programmed necrosis induced by asbestos in human mesothelial cells causes high-mobility group box 1 protein release and resultant inflammation. Proc Natl Acad Sci U S A 2010;107(28):12611-6.

[62] Teta D. Adipokines as uremic toxins. J Ren Nutr 2012;22(1):81-5.

[63] Duranton F, Cohen G, De Smet R, Rodriguez M, Jankowski J, Vanholder R, Argiles A. Normal and pathologic concentrations of uremic toxins. J Am Soc Nephrol 2012;23(7):1258-70.

[64] Huang JW, Yen CJ, Chiang HW, Hung KY, Tsai TJ, Wu KD. Adiponectin in peritoneal dialysis patients: a comparison with hemodialysis patients and subjects with normal renal function. Am J Kidney Dis 2004;43(6):1047-55.

[65] Fernandez-Riejos P, Najib S, Santos-Alvarez J, Martin-Romero C, Perez-Perez A, Gonzalez-Yanes C, Sanchez-Margalet V. Role of leptin in the activation of immune cells. Mediators Inflamm 2010;2010:568343.

[66] Teta D, Tedjani A, Burnier M, Bevington A, Brown J, Harris K. Glucose-containing peritoneal dialysis fluids regulate leptin secretion from 3T3-L1 adipocytes. Nephrol Dial Transplant 2005;20(7):1329-35.

[67] Leung JC, Chan LY, Tang SC, Chu KM, Lai KN. Leptin induces TGF-beta synthesis through functional leptin receptor expressed by human peritoneal mesothelial cell. Kidney Int 2006;69(11):2078-86.

[68] Ouchi N, Walsh K. A novel role for adiponectin in the regulation of inflammation. Arterioscler Thromb Vasc Biol 2008;28(7):1219-21.

[69] Huh JY, Seo EY, Lee HB, Ha H. Glucose-based peritoneal dialysis solution suppresses adiponectin synthesis through oxidative stress in an experimental model of peritoneal dialysis. Perit Dial Int 2012;32(1):20-8.

[70] Noh H, Kim JS, Han KH, Lee GT, Song JS, Chung SH, Jeon JS, Ha H, Lee HB. Oxidative stress during peritoneal dialysis: implications in functional and structural changes in the membrane. Kidney Int 2006;69(11):2022-8.

[71] Ambade A, Mandrekar P. Oxidative stress and inflammation: essential partners in alcoholic liver disease. Int J Hepatol 2012;2012:853175.

[72] Lee HB, Yu MR, Song JS, Ha H. Reactive oxygen species amplify protein kinase C signaling in high glucose-induced fibronectin expression by human peritoneal mesothelial cells. Kidney Int 2004;65(4):1170-9.

[73] Aufricht C, Endemann M, Bidmon B, Arbeiter K, Mueller T, Regele H, Herkner K, Eickelberg O. Peritoneal dialysis fluids induce the stress response in human mesothelial cells. Perit Dial Int 2001;21(1):85-8.

[74] Arbeiter K, Bidmon B, Endemann M, Bender TO, Eickelberg O, Ruffingshofer D, Mueller T, Regele H, Herkner K, Aufricht C. Peritoneal dialysate fluid composition determines heat shock protein expression patterns in human mesothelial cells. Kidney Int 2001;60(5):1930-7.

[75] Boehm M, Bergmeister H, Kratochwill K, Vargha R, Lederhuber H, Aufricht C. Cellular stress-response modulators in the acute rat model of peritoneal dialysis. Pediatr Nephrol 2010;25(1):169-72.

[76] Bender TO, Riesenhuber A, Endemann M, Herkner K, Witowski J, Jorres A, Aufricht C. Correlation between HSP-72 expression and IL-8 secretion in human mesothelial cells. Int J Artif Organs 2007;30(3):199-203.

[77] Jameson JM, Cauvi G, Sharp LL, Witherden DA, Havran WL. Gammadelta T cell-induced hyaluronan production by epithelial cells regulates inflammation. J Exp Med 2005;201(8):1269-79.

[78] Nathan C. Points of control in inflammation. Nature 2002;420(6917):846-52.

[79] Yung S, Coles GA, Williams JD, Davies M. The source and possible significance of hyaluronan in the peritoneal cavity. Kidney Int 1994;46(2):527-33.

[80] Yung S, Thomas GJ, Stylianou E, Williams JD, Coles GA, Davies M. Source of peritoneal proteoglycans. Human peritoneal mesothelial cells synthesize and secrete mainly small dermatan sulfate proteoglycans. Am J Pathol 1995;146(2):520-9.

[81] Jiang D, Liang J, Noble PW. Hyaluronan as an immune regulator in human diseases. Physiol Rev 2011;91(1):221-64.

[82] Jiang D, Liang J, Fan J, Yu S, Chen S, Luo Y, Prestwich GD, Mascarenhas MM, Garg HG, Quinn DA, Homer RJ, Goldstein DR, Bucala R, Lee PJ, Medzhitov R, Noble PW. Regulation of lung injury and repair by Toll-like receptors and hyaluronan. Nat Med 2005;11(11):1173-9.

[83] Schaefer L, Babelova A, Kiss E, Hausser HJ, Baliova M, Krzyzankova M, Marsche G, Young MF, Mihalik D, Gotte M, Malle E, Schaefer RM, Grone HJ. The matrix component biglycan is proinflammatory and signals through Toll-like receptors 4 and 2 in macrophages. J Clin Invest 2005;115(8):2223-33.

[84] Hildebrand A, Romaris M, Rasmussen LM, Heinegard D, Twardzik DR, Border WA, Ruoslahti E. Interaction of the small interstitial proteoglycans biglycan, decorin and fibromodulin with transforming growth factor beta. Biochem J 1994;302 (Pt 2): 527-34.

[85] Tufvesson E, Westergren-Thorsson G. Tumour necrosis factor-alpha interacts with biglycan and decorin. FEBS Lett 2002;530(1-3):124-8.

[86] Brauner A, Hylander B, Wretlind B. Tumor necrosis factor-alpha, interleukin-1 beta, and interleukin-1 receptor antagonist in dialysate and serum from patients on continuous ambulatory peritoneal dialysis. Am J Kidney Dis 1996;27(3):402-8.

[87] van de Veerdonk FL, Netea MG, Dinarello CA, Joosten LA. Inflammasome activation and IL-1beta and IL-18 processing during infection. Trends Immunol 2011;32(3): 110-6.

[88] Netea MG, Simon A, van de Veerdonk F, Kullberg BJ, Van der Meer JW, Joosten LA. IL-1beta processing in host defense: beyond the inflammasomes. PLoS Pathog 2010;6(2):e1000661.

[89] Petrilli V, Dostert C, Muruve DA, Tschopp J. The inflammasome: a danger sensing complex triggering innate immunity. Curr Opin Immunol 2007;19(6):615-22.

[90] Babelova A, Moreth K, Tsalastra-Greul W, Zeng-Brouwers J, Eickelberg O, Young MF, Bruckner P, Pfeilschifter J, Schaefer RM, Grone HJ, Schaefer L. Biglycan, a dan-

ger signal that activates the NLRP3 inflammasome via toll-like and P2X receptors. J Biol Chem 2009;284(36):24035-48.

[91] Jiang D, Liang J, Noble PW. Hyaluronan in tissue injury and repair. Annu Rev Cell Dev Biol 2007;23:435-61.

[92] Yeh ET. CRP as a mediator of disease. Circulation 2004;109(21 Suppl 1):II11-4.

[93] Liuzzo G, Biasucci LM, Gallimore JR, Grillo RL, Rebuzzi AG, Pepys MB, Maseri A. The prognostic value of C-reactive protein and serum amyloid a protein in severe unstable angina. N Engl J Med 1994;331(7):417-24.

[94] Lacson E, Jr., Levin NW. C-reactive protein and end-stage renal disease. Semin Dial 2004;17(6):438-48.

[95] Pasceri V, Cheng JS, Willerson JT, Yeh ET. Modulation of C-reactive protein-mediated monocyte chemoattractant protein-1 induction in human endothelial cells by anti-atherosclerosis drugs. Circulation 2001;103(21):2531-4.

[96] Soni SS, Cruz D, Bobek I, Chionh CY, Nalesso F, Lentini P, de Cal M, Corradi V, Virzi G, Ronco C. NGAL: a biomarker of acute kidney injury and other systemic conditions. Int Urol Nephrol 2010;42(1):141-50.

[97] Bolignano D, Coppolino G, Lacquaniti A, Buemi M. From kidney to cardiovascular diseases: NGAL as a biomarker beyond the confines of nephrology. Eur J Clin Invest 2010;40(3):273-6.

[98] Li FK, Davenport A, Robson RL, Loetscher P, Rothlein R, Williams JD, Topley N. Leukocyte migration across human peritoneal mesothelial cells is dependent on directed chemokine secretion and ICAM-1 expression. Kidney Int 1998;54(6):2170-83.

[99] Fain JN, Madan AK. Regulation of monocyte chemoattractant protein 1 (MCP-1) release by explants of human visceral adipose tissue. Int J Obes (Lond) 2005;29(11): 1299-307.

[100] Takayama F, Miyazaki T, Aoyama I, Tsukushi S, Sato M, Yamazaki C, Shimokata K, Niwa T. Involvement of interleukin-8 in dialysis-related arthritis. Kidney Int 1998;53(4):1007-13.

[101] Tekstra J, Visser CE, Tuk CW, Brouwer-Steenbergen JJ, Burger CW, Krediet RT, Beelen RH. Identification of the major chemokines that regulate cell influxes in peritoneal dialysis patients. J Am Soc Nephrol 1996;7(11):2379-84.

[102] Lai KN, Lam MF, Leung JC, Chan LY, Lam CW, Chan IH, Chan HW, Li CS, Wong SS, Ho YW, Cheuk A, Tong MK, Tang SC. A study of the clinical and biochemical profile of peritoneal dialysis fluid low in glucose degradation products. Perit Dial Int 2012;32(3):280-91.

[103] Lai KN, Leung JC. Peritoneal adipocytes and their role in inflammation during peritoneal dialysis. Mediators Inflamm 2010;2010:495416.

[104] Kajiyama H, Shibata K, Ino K, Nawa A, Mizutani S, Kikkawa F. Possible involvement of SDF-1alpha/CXCR4-DPPIV axis in TGF-beta1-induced enhancement of migratory potential in human peritoneal mesothelial cells. Cell Tissue Res 2007;330(2):221-9.

[105] Papagianni A, Kokolina E, Kalovoulos M, Vainas A, Dimitriadis C, Memmos D. Carotid atherosclerosis is associated with inflammation, malnutrition and intercellular adhesion molecule-1 in patients on continuous ambulatory peritoneal dialysis. Nephrol Dial Transplant 2004;19(5):1258-63.

[106] Wang AY, Lam CW, Wang M, Woo J, Chan IH, Lui SF, Sanderson JE, Li PK. Circulating soluble vascular cell adhesion molecule 1: relationships with residual renal function, cardiac hypertrophy, and outcome of peritoneal dialysis patients. Am J Kidney Dis 2005;45(4):715-29.

[107] Barrington R, Zhang M, Fischer M, Carroll MC. The role of complement in inflammation and adaptive immunity. Immunol Rev 2001;180:5-15.

[108] Tang S, Leung JC, Chan LY, Tsang AW, Chen CX, Zhou W, Lai KN, Sacks SH. Regulation of complement C3 and C4 synthesis in human peritoneal mesothelial cells by peritoneal dialysis fluid. Clin Exp Immunol 2004;136(1):85-94.

[109] Mizuno T, Mizuno M, Morgan BP, Noda Y, Yamada K, Okada N, Yuzawa Y, Matsuo S, Ito Y. Specific collaboration between rat membrane complement regulators Crry and CD59 protects peritoneum from damage by autologous complement activation. Nephrol Dial Transplant 2011;26(6):1821-30.

[110] Mizuno M, Ito Y, Mizuno T, Harris CL, Suzuki Y, Okada N, Matsuo S, Morgan BP. Membrane complement regulators protect against fibrin exudation increases in a severe peritoneal inflammation model in rats. Am J Physiol Renal Physiol 2012;302(10):F1245-51.

[111] Yanez-Mo M, Lara-Pezzi E, Selgas R, Ramirez-Huesca M, Dominguez-Jimenez C, Jimenez-Heffernan JA, Aguilera A, Sanchez-Tomero JA, Bajo MA, Alvarez V, Castro MA, del Peso G, Cirujeda A, Gamallo C, Sanchez-Madrid F, Lopez-Cabrera M. Peritoneal dialysis and epithelial-to-mesenchymal transition of mesothelial cells. N Engl J Med 2003;348(5):403-13.

[112] Yang AH, Chen JY, Lin JK. Myofibroblastic conversion of mesothelial cells. Kidney Int 2003;63(4):1530-9.

[113] Gao D, Zhao ZZ, Liang XH, Li Y, Cao Y, Liu ZS. Effect of peritoneal dialysis on expression of vascular endothelial growth factor, basic fibroblast growth factor and endostatin of the peritoneum in peritoneal dialysis patients. Nephrology (Carlton) 2011;16(8):736-42.

[114] Leung JC, Chan LY, Tam KY, Tang SC, Lam MF, Cheng AS, Chu KM, Lai KN. Regulation of CCN2/CTGF and related cytokines in cultured peritoneal cells under conditions simulating peritoneal dialysis. Nephrol Dial Transplant 2009;24(2):458-69.

[115] Friedman JM. Obesity in the new millennium. Nature 2000;404(6778):632-4.

[116] Yang AH, Huang SW, Chen JY, Lin JK, Chen CY. Leptin augments myofibroblastic conversion and fibrogenic activity of human peritoneal mesothelial cells: a functional implication for peritoneal fibrosis. Nephrol Dial Transplant 2007;22(3):756-62.

[117] Teta D, Maillard M, Halabi G, Burnier M. The leptin/adiponectin ratio: potential implications for peritoneal dialysis. Kidney Int Suppl 2008(108):S112-8.

[118] Zemel D, Betjes MG, Dinkla C, Struijk DG, Krediet RT. Analysis of inflammatory mediators and peritoneal permeability to macromolecules shortly before the onset of overt peritonitis in patients treated with CAPD. Perit Dial Int 1995;15(2):134-41.

[119] Mariano F, Tetta C, Montrucchio G, Cavalli PL, Camussi G. Role of alpha 1-proteinase inhibitor in restraining peritoneal inflammation in CAPD patients. Kidney Int 1992;42(3):735-42.

[120] Clark SR, Guy CJ, Scurr MJ, Taylor PR, Kift-Morgan AP, Hammond VJ, Thomas CP, Coles B, Roberts GW, Eberl M, Jones SA, Topley N, Kotecha S, O'Donnell VB. Esterified eicosanoids are acutely generated by 5-lipoxygenase in primary human neutrophils and in human and murine infection. Blood 2011;117(6):2033-43.

[121] Morishita Y, Watanabe M, Hirahara I, Akimoto T, Muto S, Kusano E. Level of 8-OHdG in drained dialysate appears to be a marker of peritoneal damage in peritoneal dialysis. Int J Nephrol Renovasc Dis 2012;5:9-14.

[122] Hirahara I, Ogawa Y, Kusano E, Asano Y. Activation of matrix metalloproteinase-2 causes peritoneal injury during peritoneal dialysis in rats. Nephrol Dial Transplant 2004;19(7):1732-41.

[123] Nishina M, Endoh M, Suzuki D, Tanabe R, Endoh H, Hirahara I, Sakai H. Neutral-pH peritoneal dialysis solution improves peritoneal function and decreases matrix metalloproteinase-2 (MMP-2) in patients undergoing continuous ambulatory peritoneal dialysis (CAPD). Clin Exp Nephrol 2004;8(4):339-43.

[124] Hirahara I, Inoue M, Okuda K, Ando Y, Muto S, Kusano E. The potential of matrix metalloproteinase-2 as a marker of peritoneal injury, increased solute transport, or progression to encapsulating peritoneal sclerosis during peritoneal dialysis--a multicentre study in Japan. Nephrol Dial Transplant 2007;22(2):560-7.

[125] Musial K, Zwolinska D. Hsp27 as a marker of cell damage in children on chronic dialysis. Cell Stress Chaperones 2012.

[126] Alscher DM, Braun N, Biegger D, Fritz P. Peritoneal mast cells in peritoneal dialysis patients, particularly in encapsulating peritoneal sclerosis patients. Am J Kidney Dis 2007;49(3):452-61.

[127] Kondo S, Kagami S, Kido H, Strutz F, Muller GA, Kuroda Y. Role of mast cell tryptase in renal interstitial fibrosis. J Am Soc Nephrol 2001;12(8):1668-76.

[128] Cavallini N, Delbro D, Tobin G, Braide M. Neuropeptide release augments serum albumin loss and reduces ultrafiltration in peritoneal dialysis. Perit Dial Int 2012;32(2): 168-76.

[129] Bird SD, Walker RJ. Mast cell histamine-induced calcium transients in cultured human peritoneal mesothelial cells. Perit Dial Int 1998;18(6):626-36.

[130] Lai KN, Li PK, Woo KS, Lui SF, Leung JC, Law E, Nicholls MG. Vasoactive hormones in uremic patients on continuous ambulatory peritoneal dialysis. Clin Nephrol 1991;35(5):218-23.

[131] Duman S. The renin-angiotensin system and peritoneal dialysis. Perit Dial Int 2004;24(1):5-9.

[132] Nakamoto H, Imai H, Fukushima R, Ishida Y, Yamanouchi Y, Suzuki H. Role of the renin-angiotensin system in the pathogenesis of peritoneal fibrosis. Perit Dial Int 2008;28 Suppl 3:S83-7.

[133] Leung JC, Chan LY, Tang SC, Lam MF, Chow CW, Lim AI, Lai KN. Oxidative damages in tubular epithelial cells in IgA nephropathy: role of crosstalk between angiotensin II and aldosterone. J Transl Med 2011;9:169.

[134] Catalan MP, Reyero A, Egido J, Ortiz A. Acceleration of neutrophil apoptosis by glucose-containing peritoneal dialysis solutions: role of caspases. J Am Soc Nephrol 2001;12(11):2442-9.

[135] Ha H, Yu MR, Choi HN, Cha MK, Kang HS, Kim MH, Lee HB. Effects of conventional and new peritoneal dialysis solutions on human peritoneal mesothelial cell viability and proliferation. Perit Dial Int 2000;20 Suppl 5:S10-8.

[136] Jorres A, Williams JD, Topley N. Peritoneal dialysis solution biocompatibility: inhibitory mechanisms and recent studies with bicarbonate-buffered solutions. Perit Dial Int 1997;17 Suppl 2:S42-6.

[137] Hekking LH, Zareie M, Driesprong BA, Faict D, Welten AG, de Greeuw I, Schadee-Eestermans IL, Havenith CE, van den Born J, ter Wee PM, Beelen RH. Better preservation of peritoneal morphologic features and defense in rats after long-term exposure to a bicarbonate/lactate-buffered solution. J Am Soc Nephrol 2001;12(12): 2775-86.

[138] Zareie M, Keuning ED, ter Wee PM, Schalkwijk CG, Beelen RH, van den Born J. Improved biocompatibility of bicarbonate/lactate-buffered PDF is not related to pH. Nephrol Dial Transplant 2006;21(1):208-16.

[139] Furuya R, Odamaki M, Kumagai H, Hishida A. Beneficial effects of icodextrin on plasma level of adipocytokines in peritoneal dialysis patients. Nephrol Dial Transplant 2006;21(2):494-8.

[140] Martikainen T, Teppo AM, Gronhagen-Riska C, Ekstrand A. Benefit of glucose-free dialysis solutions on glucose and lipid metabolism in peritoneal dialysis patients. Blood Purif 2005;23(4):303-10.

[141] Sisca S, Maggiore U. Beneficial effect of icodextrin on the hypertriglyceridemia of CAPD patients. Perit Dial Int 2002;22(6):727-9.

[142] Martikainen T, Ekstrand A, Honkanen E, Teppo AM, Gronhagen-Riska C. Do interleukin-6, hyaluronan, soluble intercellular adhesion molecule-1 and cancer antigen 125 in dialysate predict changes in peritoneal function? A 1-year follow-up study. Scand J Urol Nephrol 2005;39(5):410-6.

[143] Moriishi M, Kawanishi H, Watanabe H, Tsuchiya S. Effect of icodextrin-based peritoneal dialysis solution on peritoneal membrane. Adv Perit Dial 2005;21:21-4.

[144] Parikova A, Zweers MM, Struijk DG, Krediet RT. Peritoneal effluent markers of inflammation in patients treated with icodextrin-based and glucose-based dialysis solutions. Adv Perit Dial 2003;19:186-90.

[145] Yang SY, Huang JW, Shih KY, Hsu SP, Chu PL, Chu TS, Wu KD. Factors associated with increased plasma homocysteine in patients using an amino acid peritoneal dialysis fluid. Nephrol Dial Transplant 2005;20(1):161-6.

[146] Martikainen TA, Teppo AM, Gronhagen-Riska C, Ekstrand AV. Glucose-free dialysis solutions: inductors of inflammation or preservers of peritoneal membrane? Perit Dial Int 2005;25(5):453-60.

[147] Williams JD, Topley N, Craig KJ, Mackenzie RK, Pischetsrieder M, Lage C, Passlick-Deetjen J. The Euro-Balance Trial: the effect of a new biocompatible peritoneal dialysis fluid (balance) on the peritoneal membrane. Kidney Int 2004;66(1):408-18.

[148] Jones S, Holmes CJ, Krediet RT, Mackenzie R, Faict D, Tranaeus A, Williams JD, Coles GA, Topley N. Bicarbonate/lactate-based peritoneal dialysis solution increases cancer antigen 125 and decreases hyaluronic acid levels. Kidney Int 2001;59(4): 1529-38.

[149] Cooker LA, Luneburg P, Holmes CJ, Jones S, Topley N. Interleukin-6 levels decrease in effluent from patients dialyzed with bicarbonate/lactate-based peritoneal dialysis solutions. Perit Dial Int 2001;21 Suppl 3:S102-7.

[150] Fusshoeller A, Plail M, Grabensee B, Plum J. Biocompatibility pattern of a bicarbonate/lactate-buffered peritoneal dialysis fluid in APD: a prospective, randomized study. Nephrol Dial Transplant 2004;19(8):2101-6.

[151] Lai KN, Leung JC. Inflammation in peritoneal dialysis. Nephron Clin Pract 2010;116(1):c11-8.

Chapter 5

The Association with Cardiovascular Events and Residual Renal Function in Peritoneal Dialysis

Betül Kalender and Necmi Eren

Additional information is available at the end of the chapter

http://dx.doi.org/10.5772/56597

1. Introduction

Life expectancy among the patients with chronic kidney disease (CKD), especially among the ones with end-stage renal disease (ESRD) has decreased that is significantly lower than the general population. The leading cause of morbidity and mortality among the dialysis patients with ESRD are cardiovascular disease (CVD) which are reported to be responsible of a 50% mortality rate in these patients [1].

The prevalence of traditional cardiovascular risk factors such as hypertension, hyperlipidemia, diabetes, physical inactivity is higher in dialysis patients. Besides these, there are uremia-specific, nontraditional risk factors, including volume overload, anemia, disordered mineral metabolism, increased inflammation and oxidative stress, and malnutrition, all of which are associated with higher all-cause and cardiovascular mortality in dialysis patients. Cardiovascular risk factors that are unique to peritoneal dialysis (PD) patients, including residual renal function (RRF), peritoneal membran integrity, infection, dialysis center size, patient education and training, all of which are also associated with higher all-cause and cardiovascular mortality in dialysis patients.

In 1995, Maiorca et al were among the first to note an independent relationship between the presence of residual renal function, and survival in patients on dialysis [2]. Several subsequent studies reported similar findings that residual renal function but not the dose of peritoneal dialysis was a powerful predictor of survival in peritoneal dialysis patients [3-7].

The mechanism underlying survival benefits associated with RRF in PD patients is not clear. RRF has been implicated to be important in maintaining the fluid balance of patients on PD. RRF also plays an important role in phosphorus control, and removal of middle molecular uremic toxins. In addition, loss of RRF is associated with higher arterial pressure, more severe anemia, greater degree of inflammation and malnutrition, and greater cardiac hypertrophy, all of which contribute to increased cardiovascular events in peritoneal dialysis patients.

The Framingham Study showed the relationship of left ventricular hypertrophy (LVH) with higher cardiovascular mortality in general population [8]. Studies showed that prevalence of LVH is higher among dialysis patients [9,10]. The severity of left ventricular hypertrophy, a strong independent predictor of mortality in patients on dialysis, inversely correlates with the presence of RRF [10]. LVH may cause cardiovascular events, such as congestive heart failure, arrhythmia, and sudden cardiac death in dialysis patients [11,12].

This chapter will review the association with cardiovascular events and residual renal function in patients on peritoneal dialysis.

2. Measurement of residual renal function

Residual renal function represents the function of the native kidneys or the in situ kidney allograft [13]. RRF may be measured or estimated. Residual GFR measured by isotope clearance is considered to be the standard measure of renal function. Other tests, such as serum creatinine, creatinine clearance, urea clearance, an average of the creatinine and urea clearances, and urine volume have been used to evaluate RRF in chronic kidney disease. The simplest measure of RRF is urine volume. Despite its shortcomings, urine volume has been correlated to GFR in studies, and most authors defined loss of RRF as estimated urine volume ≤ 200 mL/24 hour.

NKF-K/DOQI and European guidelines currently recommend that mean urea and creatinine clearance be used for PD patients [13,14]. Urine collections (24 hours for PD, interdialytic for HD) to measure urea and/or creatinine clearance could be done at baseline and every 1 to 3 months in patients with RRF.

3. Cardiovascular disease in peritoneal dialysis patients

Although dialysis technology has improved markedly over the last 20 years, dialysis patients still die at a rate of about 10–20% per year – a survival worse than that documented in patients with cancer disease [1]. Early studies observed that morbidity and mortality rates were lower in HD patients [15]. However, further studies discovered that PD could achieve patient survival that was the same or better than that with HD [16-18].

Among dialysis patients, cardiovascular disease is common, with similar cardiovascular mortality rates in a 20-year-old dialysis patient and an 80-year-old member of the general population. CVD including ischemic heart disease, left ventricular hypertrophy, heart failure, arrhythmia and sudden cardiac death, accounts for most deaths in dialysis patients (approximately 50%). Even though accelerated atherosclerosis seems to be an important cause of the high cardiovascular mortality in dialysis patients, the CVD pattern is atypical and a lot of nontraditional risk factors, such as volume expansion, anemia, inflammation, oxidative stress, malnutrition, disordered mineral metabolism, sympathetic overactivity, and loss of residual renal function contribute to the high cardiovascular mortality rate. The data of the United States Renal Data System (USRDS) registry show that cardiac arrest/arrhythmia is the major cause of cardiovascular death in this patient population [1].

Ischemic heart disease may be suboptimal diagnosis and treatment because atypical clinical manifestations in dialysis patients. Heart failure rates are also extremely high and commonly presents specific symptoms. Among the cause of deaths are cerebrovascular disease and peripheral vascular disease in dialysis patients. Arrhythmias are also extremely common in dialysis patients, most likely reflecting the prevalence of structural heart disease, ischemic heart disease, and electrolyte abnormalities.

LVH is the most prominent structural cardiovascular alteration in dialysis patients. LVH is defined as the increase in myocard fibrils and in the mass of left ventricle muscle that generally emerges as a result of a volume or pressure load [19]. There are two kinds of LVH one of which is concentric hypertrophy due to excessive pressure load and the other is eccentric hypertrophy due to volume load on left ventricle [20]. Diagnosis of LVH is readily accomplished with echocardiography in patients with symptomatic or asymptomatic cardiac diseases. A study demonstrated that 74% of ESRD patients have LVH [9]. In another study was showed that 92% of PD patients have LVH [10]. It was reported that in dialysis patients, high left ventricular mass index and cavity volume were independently associated with death after two years [9]. It was also reported that there is a tendency of heart failure or early death for the dialysis patients that have presence of LVH at the beginning of the therapy. Authors concluded that potentially reversible risk factors include anaemia, hypertension, hypoalbuminaemia and ischaemic heart disease [20].

In a prospective study in 161 dialysis patients were tested the prognostic value of changes in left ventricular mass index (LVMi) [expressed as LVM/height$^{2.71}$], on survival and incident cardiovascular events. In this purpose, echocardiography was performed twice, 18 +/- 2 SD months apart. It was found that the rate of increase of LVMi was significantly higher in patients with incident cardiovascular events than in those without such events. In their multiple Cox regression analysis, (including age, diabetes, smoking, homocysteine), showed that 1 g/m$^{2.7}$/month increase in LVMi was associated with a 62% increase in the incident risk of fatal and nonfatal cardiovascular events. Author concluded that changes in LVMi have an independent prognostic value for cardiovascular events and provide scientific support to the use of repeated echocardiographic studies for monitoring cardiovascular risk in dialysis patients [11].

A prospective study was performed by Foley et al, in eastern Canada. In 432 dialysis patients, they showed that a lowering of cardiac size and an increase in fractional shortening over a 1-year period after inception of dialysis therapy were both associated with a reduced subsequent likelihood of cardiac failure. They suggested that the associations between serial change in both left ventricular mass index and fractional shortening and subsequent cardiac failure persisted after adjusting for baseline age, diabetes, ischemic heart disease, and the corresponding baseline echocardiographic parameter. Regression of left ventricular abnormalities is associated with an improved cardiac outcome in dialysis patients [21]. In another study by

London et al. demonstrated that 10% decrease in left ventricular mass of dialysis patients leads to 28% decrease in the mortality caused by cardiovascular events [22].

Several mechanisms may contribute to explain the increased cardiovascular risk associated with LVH. LVH is associated with myocardial fibrosis, systolic and diastolic dysfunction which is an important factor in the evolution of cardiac arrhythmia and heart failure. Furthermore LVH reduces coronary reserve and induces cardiac ischemia which may in turn promote myocardial infarction and lethal arrhythmias [11]. In addition to it was showed that there is the link between uremic cardiomyopathy, QT interval and dispersal, and arrhythmias in chronic kidney disease patients [23]. It was suggessted that arrhythmias due to the abnormal electrical conduction of fibrotic ventricles can become the leading cause of mortality in dialysis patients by resulting in sudden cardiac arrest.

In summary, concentric and eccentric left ventricular hypertrophy are common and progressive disorders in dialysis patients and are associated with cardiac ischemia, cardiac failure, arrhythmias and sudden cardiac death.

4. Survival benefits of residual renal function in peritoneal dialysis

Studies have been demonstrated that the presence of RRF is associated with survival in both PD and hemodialysis (HD) patients. As mentioned above, in 1995, Maiorca et al were among the first to note an independent relationship between the presence of RRF and survival in patients on dialysis [2]. In their analysis of 102 patients on PD and HD, every 1-mL/min increase in glomerular filtration rate (GFR) was associated with a 40% reduced risk of death in the entire cohort and a 50% reduced risk of death in patients on PD.

In a prospective observational study it was performed in 1446 PD patients and weekly Kt/V urea and creatinine clearance were determined at study baseline. During the seven month period of follow-up, there were 140 deaths. It was reported that in separate logistic regression models that included all of the studied risk factors, using separate variables for the urinary and peritoneal components of dialysis adequacy, each 10 L/week/1.73 m^2 increase in the urinary component of weekly creatinine clearance was associated with a 40% decreased risk of death, and each 0.1 unit increase in the urinary component of weekly Kt/V urea was associated with a 12% decreased risk of death. In contrast, the dialysate components of neither weekly creatinine clearance nor weekly Kt/V urea were predictive of death. Other factors that were associated with an increased risk of death included increasing age, diabetes mellitus as the cause of end-stage renal disease, and a history of myocardial infarction. Authors concluded that residual renal function is an important predictor of death in peritoneal dialysis patients [3]. Another study it was conducted in 1603 PD patients. Similarly, the analysis of clearance data or peritoneal equilibration test (PET) studies also confirmed residual renal function was strongly correlated with survival, but peritoneal clearance was not [4].

Reanalysis of data from the multicenter prospective cohort Canada–United States (CANUSA) study of 680 incident patients on PD demonstrated that for each 5 L/wk per 1.73 m^2 increment in residual glomerular filtration rate (rGFR), there was a 12% decrease in the relative risk of death but no association with peritoneal creatinine clearance. It was suggested that the predictive power for mortality in patients on PD was attributed to RRF and not to the dose of PD. Moreover it has reported that low residual renal function at start of peritoneal dialysis is associated with increased mortality in patients with end-stage renal disease [5].

Similar results were found in The Netherlands Cooperative Study on the Adequacy of Dialysis (NECOSAD-2), in which each 1-ml/min increase in rGFR was associated with a 12% reduction in mortality, and peritoneal clearance had no significant effect on patient survival [6].

ADEquacy of Peritoneal Dialysis in MEXico (ADEMEX) study lent further important evidence that residual renal and peritoneal dialysis clearance are not equivalent and thus not simply additive. In this prospective randomized controlled study, increasing peritoneal clearance showed no additional impact on the survival of either all patients or anuric PD patients, but the presence of RRF has a beneficial effect on patient survival [7].

These findings has been shown that the contribution of residual renal and peritoneal dialysis clearance to the survival of peritoneal dialysis patients is not equivalent. It was also suggested that preservation of RRF has an important role in the survival of peritoneal dialysis patients.

The mechanism underlying survival benefits associated with RRF in peritoneal dialysis has been drawn very much attention. The details will be discussed in further sections.

5. Risk factors of cardiovascular disease in peritoneal dialysis patients

Dialysis patients have a high prevalance of traditional (Framingham) cardiovascular risk factors such as hypertension, left ventricular hypertrophy, hyperlipidemia, diabetes, and physical inactivity. There are several patient factors that affect survival on PD, most of which are nonmodifiable. For example, presence of diabetes, age, and ESRD etiology are all nonmodifiable independent predictors of patient survival [24].

Besides traditional cardiovascular risk factors, there are uremia-specific, nontraditional risk factors, including increased inflammation and oxidative stress, malnutrition, volume overload, anemia, and disordered mineral metabolism, all of which are associated with higher all-cause and cardiovascular mortality in dialysis patients.

In the general population, modification of traditional cardiovascular risk factors decreases morbidity and mortality. However, the benefit of modifying these traditional and also nontraditional risk factors remains unclear because randomized, placebo-controlled trials in patients with chronic kidney disease (CKD) have so far been disappointing and unable to show a survival benefit of various treatment strategies, such a lipid-lowering, increased dialysis dose and normalization of hemoglobin [25,26]. This realization has focused attention on non-traditional modifiable risk factors uniqe to the PD patients. Modifiable cardiovascular risk factors that are unique to peritoneal dialysis patients, including residual renal function, peritoneal membran integrity, infection, dialysis center size, patient education and training, all of which are also associated with higher all-cause and cardiovascular mortality in dialysis patients.

As known that inflammation is highly prevalent in patients on dialysis and established to be a powerful predictor of mortality. Studies point to the increased concentrations of acute phase reactants and proinflammatory cytokines in chronic uremia [27-29], suggesting a chronic inflammatory state in CKD patients, especially in stages 3 to 5. Wang et al, found that in patients with high CRP levels, LVMi and left ventricular end diastolic diameter were high while ejection fraction (EF) and fractional shortening were lower. In multivariable Cox regression analysis they showed that every 1 mg/L increase in high-sensitivity C-reactive protein (hsCRP) was independently predictive of higher all-cause mortality and cardiovascular mortality in PD patients. It was also found that, other significant predictors for all-cause mortality included age, gender, atherosclerotic vascular disease, LVMi and residual GFR. In addition, age, history of heart failure, atherosclerotic vascular disease, and residual GFR were also independently predictive of cardiovascular mortality. Author concluded that, a single, random hs-CRP level has significant and independent prognostic value in PD patients [30]. Although the association between inflammation and cardiovascular diseases is well established the mechanism that inflammation accelerates this process is not clear. It was suggested that inflammation plays an important role on the development and progression of atherosclerosis through endothelial dysfunction, insulin resistance and oxidative stress such as increased lipid peroxidation and depletion of antioxidants [31].

Studies demonstrated that malnutrition prevalence is 23-76% and 18-50% respectively among hemodialysis and peritoneal dialysis patients [32-35]. Malnutrition is associated with low serum albumin, transferrin and prealbumin levels. Malnutrition indicators such as serum albumin level, subjective global assessment (SGA), daily protein-calorie intake and adjusted protein catabolism rate (nPCR) are reported to be important determinants of morbidity and mortality for PD patients in many studies [36-38]. Appetite loss because of abdominal distention in PD patients may directly causes malnutrition. It was known that chronic inflammation observed in CKD patients is an important causative factor for poor nutritional status determined in these patients. The concomitance of malnutrition and inflammation had also been indicated in the pathogenesis of increased cardiovascular morbidity and mortality in dialysis patients [39]. This situation is called the syndrome of malnutrition, inflammation, atherosclerosis (MIA) [40].

Mineral metabolism disorders, such as hyperphosphatemia is prevalent in PD patients [41]. Hyperphosphatemia has been linked to vascular and valvular calcification and there is an increasing recognition of a high prevalence of vascular and valvular calcification that may contribute to the increased cardiovascular mortality in the PD patients. Risk factors for valvular diseases or calcification are mineral metabolism disorders, dialysis duration, hypoalbuminemia, inflamation and being elderly. Valvular calcification may cause conduction disorders through regurgitation or substantial stenosis (mostly at aorta valve), hiss bundle involvement that results in complete cardiac block [42]. In a study, Wang et al demonstrated that 30% of PD patients have cardiac valve calcification [43]. The same study showed that even patients' calcium phosphorus product (CaxP) levels are normal, inflammation and malnutrition can be accompanied by valvular calcification. This finding proves that in addition to the association between valvular calcification and calcium phosphorus product (CaxP), inflammation and malnutrition also contribute to the process. It is known that fetuin-A is a negative acute phase protein and inhibitor of calcification. Dervisoglu et al also found negative correlation between serum fetuin-A and cytokine concentration in CKD patients [44]. This finding support the idea of inflammation-dependent down regulation of fetuin-A expression. It is reported that, serum fetuin-A independent from high serum CRP and CaxP levels is inversely related with valvular calcification [45]. This study also demonstrated that low serum fetuin-A level is associated with valvular calcification, atherosclerosis, malnutrition, and inflammation, and it is an important determinant for fatal and non-fatal cardiovascular events and all-cause mortality. Another study by Wang et al, valvular calcification was identified as a strong and independent risk factor for cardiovascular and all-cause mortality in PD patients. Clinically mortality rates similar to patients with atherosclerotic vascular complications, indicate valvular calcification to be a form of atherosclerosis [46]. Wang et al, also found an increase in the thickness of the carotid artery intima media in addition to existing valvular calcification in PD patients [47]. Malnutrition and inflammation in ESRD patients, along with high calcium load and calcium-phosphorus imbalance may also be factors that cause valvular and vascular calcification.

It is well known that anemia is also prevalent in peritoneal dialysis patients. In many studies anemia was found to be associated with high morbidity and mortality rates in peritoneal dialysis patients. Among these studies one carried out by Li et al, studied 13,974 erythropoietin-treated Medicare patients who initiated peritoneal dialysis between 1991 and 1998. Mean hemoglobin levels for the first 6 months of the study and, subsequently, time to first hospitalization and death during a 2-year follow-up were determined. They found that mortality rates in nondiabetic patients were higher in those with hemoglobin values of <10 and ≥ 12 g/dL. Mortality rates in diabetic patients were highest in those with hemoglobin values of <10 g/dL, followed by those with levels of 10 to 10.9 g/dL, while those in the 11 to 11.9 and ≥ 12 g/dL categories had similar rates. As a conclusion they stated that, anemia is associated with hospitalization and mortality in a manner supporting current Kidney Dialysis Outcomes Quality Initiative (K/DOQI) hemoglobin targets in PD patients [48].

Inflammation, malnutrition, disordered mineral metabolism, and anemia are the most common uremia-specific, nontraditional cardiovascular risk factors. They are associated with higher all-cause and cardiovascular mortality in dialysis patients. It is therefore crucial to develop effective therapeutic strategies that may prevent and potentially reverse these cardiovascular risk factors.

6. Clinical benefits of preserving residual renal function in peritoneal dialysis and the association with cardiovascular events and residual renal function in peritoneal dialysis

Observational studies showed the superiority of PD compared with HD in preserving RRF [49,50]. The rate of decline in rGFR seems to be greatest in the first 3 months of at the beginning dialysis and falls thereafter. In a study by Jansen et al, RRF measured in ml/min/1.73 m^2 body surface area (BSA) declined from a mean of 5.8 at dialysis initiation to 2.2 after 1 year in PD patients and to 1.6 in those on HD [51].

Apart from providing small solute clearance, residual renal function contributes significantly to the overall health and well-being of patients on peritoneal dialysis. The benefits of RRF in PD extend beyond survival and there is a good evidence that it has a beneficial effect on fluid balance [52], blood pressure control [53], left ventricular hypertophy [10], hemoglobin levels [10], nutrition [54], and mineral metabolism [55].

6.1. Residual renal function, volume control, and cardiac hypertrophy

Residual renal salt and water excretion contribute substantially to the maintenance of euvolemia in PD patients with preserved RRF. It was reported that suboptimal sodium and water removal in patients on PD is associated with greater rates of all-cause hospitalization and mortality [56]. In the CANUSA study, urine volume was also a powerful predictor of survival. Every 250-mL/day urine output was associated with a 36% decrease in the RR of death [5]. In a prospective study it was performed in 25 of 37 PD patients and extracellular water (ECW) (by using sodium bromide); total body water (TBW) (by using deuterium oxide), peritoneal transport characteristics (D/P creat. ratio), rGFR (by urine collection) and CRP were assessed. It was found that rGFR was associated with lower extracellular fluid (ECF) volume [57]. In another retrospective study it was performed in 600 PD patients and PD adequacy, transport status, and multifrequency bioimpedance measurements of extracellular water to total body water (ECW/TBW) were evaluated. It was found that on their multivariate analysis %ECW/TBW was associated with age, number of antihypertensive medications, log CRP, and negatively with serum albumin and RRF. Authors concluded that overhydration as assessed by ECW/TBW is prevalent in PD patients, and is associated with loss of residual renal function, inflammation, malnutrition and hypertension [52].

Preservation of RRF may reduce or obviate the need for fluid restriction. RRF is also likely to decrease the need for volume removal with dialysis, and to help prevent the need for high glucose exchanges. With declining RRF, sodium and water removal become inadequate, leading to more volume overload and worsening of arterial hypertension [52,58], which is associated with more severe LVH [59].

A study demonstrated that arterial pulse pressure is the most significant blood pressure parameter in predicting future LVMi and change in LVMi in the general population [60]. This observation also confirmed in dialysis patients. In a study it was reported that arterial pulse pressure was independently associated with LVH in dialysis patients. Moreover, arterial pulse pressure was significantly and positively correlated with rGFR in PD patients in this study [10].

Wang et al, was also demonstrated an important association between degree of RRF and severity of LVH in PD patients. Moreover, loss of RRF is also associated with more severe anemia, greater degree of hypoalbuminemia, and higher arterial pressure, all of which are important risk factors for cardiac hypertrophy in patients on dialysis [10]. However, the association between LVH and RRF could not be fully explained by anemia, hypoalbuminemia, hypervolemia or hypertension. It was showed that in pre-dialysis patients, the decline in renal function was associated with an increase in the LVH [61]. After a successful kidney transplantation Riggato et al, demonstrated a regression in LVH [62]. Both of these observations suggest that degree of uremia and loss of RRF may be important in determining the LVH. The link between loss of residual renal function and cardiac hypertrophy may also explain that some non-dialyzable uremic toxins may be important in the progression of left ventricular hypertrophy in peritoneal dialysis patients and needs further evaluation.

6.2. Residual renal function and metabolic control

RRF plays an important role for removal of middle molecules and protein-bound solutes which are increasingly recognized as important uremic toxins. Cross-sectional and prospective studies by Bammens et al [63], and Pham et al [64], showed that the contribution of renal to total clearance of middle molecules (β2-microglobulin) and proteinbound substances (*P*-cresol, *P*-cresol sulfate, indican) was much greater than the renal contribution to total small-solute clearance. Patients with significant RRF are shown to have lower β2-microglobulin levels [65], and are thus, less prone to dialysis-associated amyloidosis [66], Bammens et al [63], also showed that with a progressive decrease in RRF, increasing the PD dose was able to compensate for loss of renal clearances of such small water-soluble solutes as urea and creatinine. However, permanent irreversible decreases were seen in the total clearance of middle molecules and protein-bound substances.

In PD patients it was found that RRF is positively and directly related to hemoglobin levels and nutrition parameters such as serum albumin and nPCR [67]. In 158 non-diabetic PD patients, Wang et al. showed that patients with better residual GFR were less anemic and had lower degree of hypoalbuminemia. Human erythropoietin levels were found higher in patients with RRF on maintenance hemodialysis and positively correlated with rGFR [68]. This finding shows that presence of RRF even in a small amount, account for considerable improvements in the degree of anemia.

Hyperphosphatemia is a common problem encountered in PD and HD patients and has been linked to vascular calcification and increased cardiovascular mortality in these patients [41,69]. A study was performed by Wang et al, in 252 prevalent Chinese PD patients. They found that, serum phosphorus levels were 5.6 mg/dL or greater in 44.0% of anuric patients versus 28.7% of patients with RRF. Their multiple regression analysis showed that residual glomerular filtration, despite an average of less than 2 mL/min/1.73 m^2, was independently associated with phosphorus control in PD patients. In this study was also showed that, residual GFR was negatively correlated with serum phosphorus and the product of calcium with phosphorus levels, indicating the contribution of the presence of RRF to the phosphate balance in such patients [70]. Dervisoglu et al, was also showed that residual GFR was associated with phosphorus control [71]. As a conclusion, after ingestion of dietary phosphorus, RRF is the most important factor in the control of serum phosphorus level in PD patients.

6.3. Residual renal function and inflammation and nutritional status

As mentioned above, inflammation and malnutrition are highly prevalent among dialysis patients and they are associated with higher all-cause and cardiovascular mortality in dialysis patients. Loss of RRF is also associated with increased inflammation and malnutrition in PD patients.

Chung et al, performed a retrospective analysis in new 117 peritoneal dialysis patients with initial assessments for RRF and serum CRP. It was found that patients with low RRF were older and had a higher prevalence of high CRP. In their multiple regression analysis, age and RRF were identified as factors affecting inflammation. Overall patient survival was significantly lower in the patients with low RRF, with high CRP. Authors concluded that these results indicate that in patients starting PD, low initial RRF is associated with inflammation, and low RRF and inflammation are both associated with high overall mortality [72]. In a prospective observational study, it was conducted a cohort of 160 PD patients with a mean follow-up of 35 +/- 16 (SD) months. At baseline, echocardiography and standard clinical and biochemical analyses and markers of inflammation such as circulating soluble vascular cell adhesion molecule 1(sVCAM-1) and CRP were performed in all patients. Serum sVCAM-1 levels were elevated in PD patients and showed a negative correlation with rGFR but a positive correlation with LVMi. Furthermore, patients with both sVCAM-1 and CRP levels elevated at the 50th percentile or greater were associated with the greatest death and fatal and nonfatal cardiovascular event rates [73]. In similar, using high-sensitivity C-reactive protein (hsCRP), tumor necrosis factor-alpha (TNF-alpha), interleukin-6 (IL-6), as markers of inflammation a study indicated that a low GFR is also associated with an higher inflammatory state [74].

Conversely, inflammation may exert negative effects on RRF. For example, in a retrospective analysis it was performed in 80 patients to identify risk factors influencing the decline of RRF after the initiation of peritoneal dialysis. It was found that the only independent risk factor for the decline of RRF was the rate of peritonitis by linear multiple regression analysis. This observation suggest that the presence of inflammation may accelerate the decline of RRF [75]. The exact mechanism of the relationship between residual renal function and inflammation are not clear. Although, more inflammation may have had a greater tendency to a decrease in RRF, it also is possible that loss of RRF may enhance inflammatory response and impaire cytokine clearance.

The impact of RRF on nutritional status in dialysis patients has also studied in some studies. Markers of nutritional status, such as subjective global assessment, lean body mass, and handgrip strength, all correlate with RRF in PD patients. Wang et al, performed a cross-sectional study on 242 PD patients. Appetite, dietary protein, and total calorie intake assessed by using food questionnaires appear to be enhanced in the presence of RRF. Authors was concluded that this study confirmed significant and independent effect of RRF, on dietary intake, and other nutrient intake in PD patients [76]. These may relate to the enhanced renal elimination of appetite-suppressing cytokines and liberalization of diet in the face of preserved RRF also may explain the increases in dietary intake. Another prospective observational study was conducted a cohort of 251 PD patients with a mean follow-up of 28.7 ± 14.3 months. Resting energy expenditure (REE) was measured at study baseline using indirect calorimetry together with other clinical, nutritional, and dialysis parameters. Anuric PD patients have been shown to have greater resting energy expenditure compared with patients with RRF. Using multiple regression analysis, adjusted REE was negatively associated with rGFR and serum albumin and positively associated with diabetes, cardiovascular disease, and CRP. At 2 year, the overall survival was 63.3, 73.6, and 95.9%, and cardiovascular event-free survival was 72.3, 84.6, and 97.2%, respectively, for patients in the upper, middle, and lower tertiles of REE. The significance of REE in predicting mortality was gradually reduced when additional adjustment was made for CRP, serum albumin, and rGFR in a stepwise manner. Author concluded that a higher REE is associated with increased mortality and cardiovascular death in PD patients and is partly related to its close correlations with residual kidney function, cardiovascular disease, inflammation, and malnutrition in these patients [77]. In patients on PD, it was also shown that patients without RRF had lower nPCR and serum albumin levels than their total weekly clearance (Kt/V) equal counterparts [78]. In another cross- sectional and multicenteric study, it was shown that the loss of renal function is associated with anorexia and symptoms of severe malnutrition in PD patients [79]. In a study it was also found that RRF was positively correlated with nutrition markers and negatively correlated with CRP. Moreover, as compared with patients without inflammation, patients with inflammation had significantly lower hemoglobin, serum prealbumin levels, and serum transferrin levels and a higher erythropoietin resistance index [54].

In summary, these findings suggested that loss of residual renal function contributes significantly to inflammation and malnutrition in peritoneal dialysis patients.

As mentioned above, LVH starts in early CKD, is present in 75% of patients entering dialysis, and is progressive thereafter. LVH is perhaps the most powerful indicator of cardiovascular events and mortality in patients with dialysis patients. Studies reported that the presence and progression of LVH was strongly linked to subsequent cardiovascular events and mortality in dialysis patients [11,21].

In 2002, Wang et al, were among the first to note an inversely relationship between the presence of RRF and LVH. A cross-sectional study was performed with LVMi, determined in 158 non-diabetic PD patients using echocardiography and its relationship with rGFR, and other known risk factors for LVH was evaluated. Only 12 patients had no LVH. The remaining 146 patients were stratified three groups according to the LVMi. Across the four groups of patients with increasing LVMi, there was significant decline in RRF. Patients with better-preserved RRF were less anemic and hypoalbuminemic and had a trend toward lower systolic blood pressure and arterial pulse pressure. Multiple regression analysis showed that other than age, gender, body weight, arterial pulse pressure, hemoglobin and serum albumin, known factors for LVH, RRF was also independently associated with LVMi [10]. In a recent prospective observational study with 2 years of follow-up, it was conducted a cohort of 156 PD patients with a mean follow-up of 19.2 ± 6.4 months. At baseline, echocardiography and standard clinical and biochemical analyses were performed in all patients and in 28 healthy subjects. During the follow-up period, 25 of the patients (16.0%) died, and 10 of those deaths had CV causes. Nonfatal CV events occurred in 15 patients. In the fully adjusted multivariate Cox regression analysis (co-variates: age, sex, albumin, hemoglobin, diabetes mellitus, comorbid CVD, LVMi, rGFR, dialysate-to-plasma ratio of creatinine, Kt/V urea, left ventricular ejection fraction, duration of dialysis, smoking), aortic stiffness index beta independently predicted fatal and nonfatal CV events, but not all-cause mortality. Moreover, all-cause mortality was predicted by age, serum albumin, and LVMi. Increases in age and in LVMi increased the risk of all-case mortality, but increases in serum albumin reduced that risk [80].

Wang et al, also performed a prospective study in 240 PD (39% being completely anuric) patients. It was found that the overall 2 year patient survival was 89.7 and 65.0 % for patients with preserved RRF and anuric patients, respectively. Compared with patients with preserved RRF, anuric patients were dialysed for longer, were more anaemic, and had higher calcium-phosphorus product, higher CRP, lower serum albumin, greater prevalence of malnutrition and more severe cardiac hypertrophy at baseline. Using multivariable Cox regression analysis, serum albumin, left ventricular mass index and residual GFR were significant factors associated with mortality in patients with RRF, while increasing age, atherosclerotic vascular disease and higher CRP were associated with greater mortality in anuric PD patients [55].

In another prospective observational study it was performed in 231 PD patients and LVMi, rGFR, CRP, hemoglobin, and serum albumin were determined at study baseline and related to outcomes. After follow-up for 30±14 month, 34.2% patients had died. CRP, RRF, and LVMi each were significantly predictive of all-cause mortality and cardiovascular death. Authors concluded that inflammation, RRF, and LVH are interrelated and combine adversely to increase mortality and cardiovascular death risk of PD patients [81].

Szeto et al, also performed a retrospective review to study the cause of death of 296 PD patients over a 7 year period, and compared the mortality and distribution of cause of death between patients with and without residual renal function. As expected, they found that, there was a higher proportion of vascular deaths in patients with pre-existing cardiovascular disease than those without (61.5 vs 40.6%). In addition, when patients with and without pre-existing cardiovascular disease were analysed separately, patients without pre-existing cardiovascular disease more commonly died of vascular disease after they become anuric (47.4 vs 34%). More importantly, for patients with pre-existing cardiovascular disease, there was no significant difference in the distribution of cause of death between those with and without RRF. As a result, they stated that, anuric patients had a higher mortality (nearly 50%) than those with preserved residual renal function, vascular disease was a more common cause of death in anuric patients than those with RRF (55.3 vs 40.8%). The difference was largely explained by the higher prevalence of sudden cardiac death in anuric patients (39 in 149 cases vs 19 in 147 cases) [82].

Ateş et al, performed a prospective study in 125 PD patients. Patients were monitored for three years from the beginning of the treatment. The effects of comorbidity, blood pressure, blood biochemistry, peritoneal membrane transport characteristics, Kt/V(urea), total creatinine clearance (TCC), RRF, and removal of sodium and fluid on mortality were evaluated. It was found that comorbidity, hypertensive status, serum creatinine, and total sodium and fluid removals were independent factors affecting survival in the Cox model. It was also demonstrated that RRF has a major impact on patient survival. It was also reported that Kt/V(urea) or TCC did not affect the adjusted survivals. Authors concluded that adequate fluid and sodium balance is crucial for the management of patients on PD. It was also suggested that RRF may have an important impact on the ability to maintain sodium and fluid balance in PD patients [56].

Both of these observations suggest that loss of RRF may be important in determining the LVH and subsequent cardiovascular events and mortality in dialysis patients.

7. Preservation of residual renal function

Both volume expansion and the high urea load per nephron are rapidly reversed by dialysis of any form. Therefore, many patients have a marked reduction in, or even cessation of, urine output when dialysis is instituted [83]. Peritoneal dialysis and hemodialysis may have different effects on residual renal function. As mentioned above, RRF is preserved longer in peritoneal dialysis than hemodialysis patients, but data from prospective randomized trials are lacking [49,50]. Potential reasons for RRF preservation in PD are related to better hemodynamic stability with PD that may minimize ischemic renal insults and avoidance of the extracorporeal circulation of HD that activates nephrotoxic inflammatory mediators during treatments and subsequent kidney injury [51,84,85]. However the use of ultrapure water and biocompatible membranes during HD have been shown to slow the loss of RRF in incident patients on HD [86,87]. Use of PD as an initial dialysis modality in patients with RRF has been suggested as strategy to maximize RRF preservation and, thus, survival for patients on dialysis.

Some studies suggested that automated forms of peritoneal dialysis (APD) might be associated with a more rapid decline in residual renal function and was hypothesized to be related to less stable fluid and osmotic load together with intermittent nature of APD. Other studies have found minimal effect of PD modality on the loss of residual renal function [88-91].

The newer biocompatible peritoneal dialysis solutions may slow the decline in RRF in peritoneal dialysis patients. In a multicenter, open, randomized, prospective study with a crossover design and parallel arms, a conventional, acidic, lactate-buffered fluid was compared with a pH neutral, lactate-buffered, low glucose degradation products (GDP) fluid (balance). It was concluded that the balance solution, a neutral pH, low GDP fluid, results in an improvement in local peritoneal homeostasis, as well as having a positive impact on systemic parameters, including circulating advanced glycosylation end products (AGE) and RRF [92]. In another randomized controlled study was conducted comparing use of biocompatible with standard solutions in 93 incident PD patients during a 1-year period. At 3 and 12 months, 24-hour urine samples were collected to measure volume and the mean of urea and creatinine clearance normalized to body surface area. It was demonstrated that changes in the normalized mean urea and creatinine clearance were the same for both groups, with no significant differences in secondary end points. Author concluded that the newer biocompatible solutions have not any clinically significant advantages [93]. Similarly, apparently conflicting results are present with the use of icodextrin in PD [94-96].

Loop diuretics appear beneficial in increasing urine and sodium excretion and improve fluid balance in dialysis patients with RRF, but there is so far no evidence that it preserves residual renal function. It was found that, the use of furosemide in a randomized trial of patients on PD, has no significant detrimental or beneficial effect on RRF [97]. Diuretics are likely to decrease the need for volume removal with dialysis, and to help prevent the need for high glucose exchanges.

Blockade of the renin–angiotensin system by angiotensin-converting enzyme inhibition or angiotensin receptor antagonism is a well-known approach for nephroprotection in pre-dialysis chronic kidney disease patients. The angiotensin-converting enzyme (ACE) inhibitors or angiotensin receptor blockers (ARBs) may also slow the decline in residual renal function in peritoneal dialysis patients. Li et al, was performed a study in 60 peritoneal dialysis patients who were randomly assigned to ramipril (5 mg/day) or no treatment. It was found that the average rGFR at one year was significantly higher among those given ramipril (1.72 and 0.64 mL/min per 1.73 m^2) [98]. Similar benefits in terms of preserving residual renal function have been observed with an angiotensin II receptor blocker. Suzuki et al, was also performed a randomized two-year controlled study in 34 peritoneal dialysis patients [99]. It was observed that valsartan maintained residual renal function (3.2 mL/min per 1.73 m^2 at baseline to 4.3 mL/min per 1.73 m^2) and total clearance (42.1 to 48.3 L/week per 1.73 m^2); compared with the control group, residual renal function decreased (5.9 to 2.8 mL/min per 1.73 m^2) and total clearance declined (47.1 to 31.4 L/week per 1.73 m^2). Significant differences between the two groups in terms of RRF were noted at two-year study end. These findings led the 2006 K/DOQI work group for peritoneal dialysis adequacy to recommend the use of ACE inhibitors and/or ARBs for the treatment of hypertension in patients who have RRF, because these agents may help decrease the decline in residual renal function [13]. They suggest that such agents should also be considered for nephroprotection among normotensive peritoneal dialysis patients. However, at present, there is not enough evidence to recommend the use of these agents in normotensive patients, unless they have other specific indications for these medications (such as heart failure).

The most importance strategy for preservation of RRF is avoidance of hypovolemia in peritoneal dialysis patients. Data from Netherlands Cooperative Study on the Adequacy of Dialysis study suggest that episodes hypovolemia were an independent risk factor for the loss of RRF in peritoneal dialysis patients [6]. But some authors believed that there is a cause-effect relationship between volume overload and preserving RRF in peritoneal dialysis patients. For example, Gunal et al, applied strict volume control with strong dietary salt restriction alone or combined with increased ultrafiltration (UF) in 47 peritoneal dialysis patients. Cardiothoracic index (CTI) on the chest radiograph was used as a measure of volume control. It was demonstrated that CTI decreased from 48.0% +/- 5.6% to 42.9% +/- 4.5% in 37 patients. In 19 patients who had residual renal function, 24-hour urine volume decreased to 28% of the pretreatment volume, accompanied by a mean decrease in Kt/V urea from 2.06 +/- 0.5 to 1.85 +/- 0.4 [100].

Aminoglycosides have been proven to be an efficacious treatment for peritonitis in peritoneal dialysis patients for many years. However, with the increasing emphasis on preserving residual renal function, there has been concern about the nephrotoxic potential of these compounds. However, some studies have found no effect of aminoglycoside use on the decline of RRF. In a study, preperitonitis and postperitonitis RRF were determined for 70 peritonitis episodes treated with the aminoglycoside-based regimen, 61 episodes treated without aminoglycosides, and 74 control patients without peritonitis. There was no evidence of an accelerated decline in RRF when using an empirical regimen containing aminoglycosides for peritonitis [101]. In another retrospective study it was also demonstrated that the change in residual renal function over time was similar in 1075 patients who treated with the aminoglycoside-based regimen for peritonitis as compared with 339 who did not [102].

In similar, with the increasing emphasis on preserving residual renal function, there has also been concern about the nephrotoxic potential of iodinated radiocontrast agents. In one prospective study, the RRF was evaluated at baseline and two weeks after contrast administration in 36 peritoneal dialysis patients and 36 control patients also underwent determination of RRF two weeks apart. In the contrast group, the study was performed with adequate prehydration and a minimum dose of contrast medium. Compared with baseline values, RRF and daily urine volume were not found to be significantly different 2 weeks after contrast. Following contrast, variations in RRF and daily urine volume were found to be comparable with those of the control group [103]. In a study of 10 peritoneal dialysis patients who received non-ionic hypo-osmolar contrast media, RRF (calculated as the average of renal creatinine and renal urea clearance) was measured on the day before the intervention (baseline), on days 1-7, day 10 and day 30 after intervention. It was observed a temporary decline of residual renal function after administration of contrast media, but on day 30, residual renal function were not significantly different from baseline [104]. But authors concluded that, non-ionic hypo-osmolar contrast media should be given to PD patients with the lowest possible dose and only if there is a real clinical indication.

In summary, strategies for preservation of RRF are avoidance of hypovolemia, avoidance of nephrotoxic drugs and agents (such as radiocontrast agents, nonsteroidal antiinflammatory drugs or aminoglycosides), the use of high dose of loop diuretics and the use of an ACE inhibitors or ARBs.

8. Conclusion

Residual renal function contributes significantly to the overall health and well-being of patients on PD. RRF has been implicated to be important in maintaining the fluid balance of patients on PD. RRF also plays an important role in phosphorus control, and removal of middle molecular uremic toxins. In addition, loss of RRF is associated with higher arterial pressure, more severe anemia, greater degree of inflammation and malnutrition. More importantly, loss of residual renal function is associated with greater degree LVH and more subsequent cardiovascular events and higher mortality in peritoneal dialysis patients. The contribution of residual renal and peritoneal dialysis clearance to the survival of peritoneal dialysis patients is not equivalent. Furthermore the loss of RRF may not be simply replaced by increasing peritoneal dialysis dose. It is therefore crucial to develop effective therapeutic strategies that may preserve RRF in peritoneal dialysis patients.

Author details

Betül Kalender[1*] and Necmi Eren[2]

*Address all correspondence to: bkalender@hotmail.com

1 Departments of Nephrology, Faculty of Medicine, University of Kocaeli, Turkey

2 Departments of Nephrology, Faculty of Medicine, University of Adiyaman, Turkey

References

[1] U.S. Renal Data System. USRDS 2008 Annual Data Report: Atlas of Chronic Kidney Disease and End-Stage Renal Disease in the United States. Bethesda, Md: National Institutes of Health, National Institute of Diabetes and Digestive and Kidney Diseases; 2008.

[2] Maiorca R, Brunori G, Zubani R, Cancarini GC, Manili L, Camerini C, Movilli E, Pola A, d'Avolio G, Gelatti U. Predictive value of dialysis adequacy and nutritional indices for mortality and morbidity in CAPD and HD patients. A longitudinal study. Nephrol Dial Transplant 1995;10: 2295-2305.

[3] Rocco M, Soucie JM, Pastan S, McClellan WM. Peritoneal dialysis adequacy and risk of death. Kidney Int 2000;58: 446-457.

[4] Diaz-Buxo JA, Lowrie EG, Lew NL, Zhang SM, Zhu X, Lazarus JM. Associates of mortality among peritoneal dialysis patients with special reference to peritoneal transport rates and solute clearance. Am J Kidney Dis 1999;33(3): 523-534.

[5] Bargman JM, Thorpe KE, Churchill DN and the CANUSA peritoneal dialysis study group. Relative contribution of residual renal function and peritoneal clearance to adequacy of dialysis: a reanalysis of the CANUSA study. J Am Soc Nephrol 2001;12: 2158-2162.

[6] Termorshuizen F, Korevaar JC, Dekker FW, van Manen JG, Boeschoten EW, Krediet RT; NECOSAD Study Group. The relative importance of residual renal function compared with peritoneal clearance for patient survival and quality of life: an analysis of the Netherlands Cooperative Study on the Adequacy of Dialysis (NECOSAD)-2. Am J Kidney Dis 2003;41(6): 1293-1302.

[7] Paniagua R, Amato D, Vonesh E, Correa-Rotter R, Ramos A, Moran J, Mujais S; Mexican Nephrology Collaborative Study Group. Effects of increased peritoneal clearances on mortality rates in peritoneal dialysis: ADEMEX, a prospective, randomized, controlled trial. J Am Soc Nephrol 2002;13: 1307-1320.

[8] Levy D, Garrison RJ, Savage DD, Kannel WB, Castelli WP. Prognostic implication of echocardioraphically determined left ventricular mass in the Framingham Heart Study. N Engl J Med 1999; 322: 1561-1566.

[9] Foley RN, Parfrey PS, Harnett JD, Kent GM, Martin CJ, Murray DC, Barre PE. Clinical and echocardiographic disease in patients starting end-stage renal disease therapy. Kidney Int 1995; 47: 186-192.

[10] Wang AY, Wang M, Woo J, Law MC, Chow KM, Li PK, Lui SF, Sanderson JE. A novel association between residual renal function and left ventricular hypertrophy in peritoneal dialysis patients. Kidney Int 2002;62: 639-647.

[11] Zoccali C, Benedetto FA, Mallamaci F, Tripepi G, Giacone G, Stancanelli B, Cataliotti A, Malatino LS. Left ventricular mass monitoring in the follow-up of dialysis patients: prognostic value of left ventricular hypertrophy progression. Kidney Int 2004;65(4): 1492-1498.

[12] Zoccali C, Benedetto FA, Mallamaci F, Tripepi G, Giacone G, Cataliotti A, Seminara G, Stancanelli B, Malatino LS. Prognositc value of echocardiographic indicators of left ventricular systolic function in asymptomatic dialysis patients. J Am Soc Nephrol 2004;15(4): 1029-1037.

[13] Clinical practice guidelines for peritoneal dialysis adequacy. Peritoneal Dialysis Adequacy Work Group. Am J Kidney Dis 2006;48(1): 98-129.

[14] European Best Practice Guidelines Expert Group on Hemodialysis, European Renal Association:Section I. Measurement of renal function, when to refer and when to start dialysis. Nephrol Dial Transplant 2002;17: 7-15.

[15] Bloembergen WE, Port FK, Mauger EA, Wolfe RA. A comparison of mortality between patients treated with hemodialysis and peritoneal dialysis. J Am Soc Nephrol 1995;6: 177-183.

[16] Fenton SS, Schaubel DE, Desmeules M, Morrison HI, Mao Y, Copleston P, Jeffery JR, Kjellstrand CM. Hemodialysis versus peritoneal dialysis: a comparison of adjusted mortality rates. Am J Kidney Dis 1997;30(3): 334-342.

[17] Heaf JG, Lokkegaard H, Madsen M. Initial survival advantage of peritoneal dialysis relative to haemodialysis. Nephrol Dial Transplant 2002;17(1): 112-117.

[18] Termorshuizen F, Korevaar JC, Dekker FW, Van Manen JG, Boeschoten EW, Krediet RT; Netherlands Cooperative Study on the Adequacy of Dialysis Study Group. Hemodialysis and peritoneal dialysis: comparison of adjusted mortality rates according to the duration of dialysis: analysis of The Netherlands Cooperative Study on the Adequacy of Dialysis 2. J Am Soc Nephrol 2003;14(11): 2851-2860.

[19] Goldberger AL. Electrocardiographic diagnosis of left ventricular hypertrophy. http://www.uptodate.com/index/ (accessed 12 August 2012).

[20] Parfrey PS, Foley RN, Harnett JD, Kent GM, Murray DC, Barre PE. Outcome and risk factors for left ventricular disorders in chronic uremia. Nephrol Dial Transplant 1996;11: 1277-1285.

[21] Foley RN, Parfrey PS, Kent GM, Harnett JD, Murray DC, Barre PE. Serial change in echocardiographic parameters and cardiac failure in end-stage renal disease. J Am Soc Nephrol 2000;11(5): 912-916.

[22] London GM, Pannier B, Guerin AP, Blacher J, Marchais SJ, Darne B, Metivier F, Adda H, Safar ME. Alterations of left ventricular hypertrophy in and survival of patients receiving hemodialysis: Follow up of an interventional study. J Am Soc Nephrol 2001;12: 2759-2767.

[23] Stewart GA, Gansevoort RT, Mark PB, Rooney E, McDonagh TA, Dargie HJ, Stuart R, Rodger C, Jardine AG. Electrocardiographic abnormalities and uremic cardiomyopathy. Kidney Int 2005;67: 217-226.

[24] Mujais S, Story K. Peritoneal dialysis in the US: Evaluation of outcomes in contemporary cohorts. Kidney Int Suppl 2006;103: 21-26.

[25] Kendrick J, Chonchol MB. Nontraditional risk factors for cardiovascular disease in patients with chronic kidney disease. Nat Clin Pract Nephrol 2008;4: 672-681.

[26] Stenvinkel P, Carrero JJ, Axelsson J, Lindholm B, Heimbürger O, Massy Z. Emerging biomarkers for evaluating cardiovascular risk in the chronic kidney disease patient: how do new pieces fit into the uremic puzzle? Clin J Am Soc Nephrol 2008;3(2): 505-521.

[27] Okhuma T, Minagawa T, Takada N, Ohno M, Oda H, Ohadhi H. C-reactive protein, Lipoprotein(a), and male sex contribute to carotid atherosclerosis in peritoneal dialysis patients. Am J Kidney Dis 2003;42: 355-361.

[28] Kalender B, Ozdemir AC, Koroglu G. Association of depresion with markers of nutrition and inflammation in chronic kidney disease and end-stage renal disease. Nephron Clin Pract 2006;102: 115-121.

[29] Kir HM, Eraldemir C, Dervisoglu E, Caglayan C, Kalender B. Effects of chronic kidney disease and type of dialysis on serum levels of adiponectin, TNF-alpha and high sensitive C-reactive protein. Clin Lab 2012;58(5-6): 495-500.

[30] Wang AY, Woo J, Lam CW, Wang M, Sea MM, Lui SF, Li PK, Sanderson J. Is a single time point C-reactive protein predictive of outcome in peritoneal dialysis patients? J Am Soc Nephrol 2003; 14: 1871-1879.

[31] Ozden M, Maral H, Akaydin D, Cetinalp P, Kalender B. Erythrocyte glutathione peroxidase activity, plasma malondialdehyde and erythrocyte glutathione levels in hemodialysis and CAPD patients. Clin Biochem. 2002;35(4): 269-273.

[32] Qureshi AR, Alvestrand A, Danielsson A, Divino-Filho JC, Gutierrez A, Lindholm B, Bergström J. Factors influencing malnutrition in hemodialysis patients. A cross-sectional study. Kidney Int 1998;53: 773-782.

[33] Bergstrom J, Lindholm B. Nutrition and adequacy of dialysis. How do hemodialysis and CAPD compare? Kidney Int 1993;34: 39-50.

[34] Kalender B, Dervisoglu E, Sengul E, Ozdemir AC, Akhan SC, Yalug I, Uzun H. Depression, nutritional status, and serum cytokines in peritoneal dialysis patients: is there a relationship? Perit Dial Int 2007;27: 593-595.

[35] Dervişoğlu E, Eraldemir C, Kalender B, Kır HM, Çağlayan Ç. Adipocytokines; Leptin, Adiponectin and measures of malnutrition-inflammation in chronic renal failure: is there a relationship? J Ren Nutr 2008;18: 332-337.

[36] Adequacy of dialysis and nutrition in continuous peritoneal dialysis: association with clinical outcomes. Canada-USA (CANUSA) Peritoneal Dialysis Study Group. J Am Soc Nephrol 1996;7: 198-207.

[37] Leinig CE, Moraes T, Ribeiro S, Riella MC, Olandoski M, Martins C, Pecoits-Filho R. Predictive value of malnutrition markers for mortality in peritoneal dialysis patients. J Ren Nutr 2011;21(2): 176-183.

[38] Dong J, Li Y, Xu Y, Xu R. Daily protein intake and survival in patients on peritoneal dialysis. Nephrol Dial Transplant 2011 ;26(11): 3715-3721.

[39] Kalantar-Zadeh K, Ikizler TA, Block G, Avram MM, Kopple JD. Malnutrition-inflammation complex syndrome in dialysis patients: causes and consequences. Am J Kidney Dis 2003;42: 864-881.

[40] Stenvinkel P, Heimbürger O, Lindholm B, Kaysen GA, Bergström J. Are there two types of malnutrition in chronic renal failure? Evidence for relationships between malnutrition, inflammation and atherosclerosis (MIA syndrome). Nephrol Dial Transplant 2000;15(7): 953-960.

[41] Yavuz A, Ersoy FF, Passadakis PS, Tam P, Evaggelos DM, Katopodis KP, Ozener C, Akçiçek F, Camsari T, Ateş K, Ataman R, Vlachojannis GJ, Dombros NA, Utaş C, Akpolat T, Bozfakioğlu S, Wu G, Karayaylali I, Arinsoy T, Stathakis CP, Yavuz M, Tsakiris DJ, Dimitriades AC, Yilmaz ME, Gültekin M, Süleymanlar G, Oreopoulos DG. Phosphorus control in peritoneal dialysis patients. Kidney Int Suppl 2008;108: 152-158.

[42] Stenvinkel P, Aman K, Ketteler M. Cardiovascular disease in chronic kidney disease. In: Floege J, Johnson RJ, Feehaly J (editors). Comprehensive Clinical Nephrology. Fourth ed. St. Louis, Missouri: Elsevier Saunders; 2010. p: 839-852.

[43] Wang AY, Woo J, Wang M, Sea MM, Ip R, Li PK. Association of inflammation and malnutrition with cardiac valve calcification in continuous ambulatory peritoneal dialysis patients. J Am Soc Nephrol 2001;12: 1927-1936.

[44] Dervisoglu E, Kir HM, Kalender B, Caglayan C, Eraldemir C. Serum fetuin-A a concentrations are inversely related to cytokine concentrations in patients with chronic renal failure. Cytokine 2008;44: 323-327.

[45] Wang AY, Woo J, Lam CW, Wang M, Chan IH, Gao P, Lui SF, Li PK, Sanderson JE. Associations of serum fetuin-A with malnutrition, inflammation, atherosclerosis and

valvular calcification syndrome and outcome in peritoneal dialysis patients. Nephrol Dial Transplant 2005;20: 1675-1685.

[46] Wang AY, Wang M, Woo J, Lam CW, Li PK, Lui SF, Sanderson JE. Cardiac valve calcification as an important predictor for all cause mortality and cardiovascular mortality in long-term peritoneal dialysis patients: a prospective study. J Am Soc Nephrol 2003;14: 159-168.

[47] Wang AY, Ho SS, Wang M, Liu EK, Ho S, Li PK, Lui SF, Sanderson JE. Cardiac valvular calcification as a marker of atherosclerosis and arterial calcification in end-stage renal disease. Arch Intern Med 2005;165: 327-332.

[48] Li S, Foley RN, Collins AJ. Anemia, hospitalization, and mortality in patients receiving peritoneal dialysis in the United States. Kidney Int 2004;65: 1864–1869.

[49] Moist LM, Port FK, Orzol SM, Young EW, Ostbye T, Wolfe RA, Hulbert-Shearon T, Jones CA, Bloembergen WE. Predictors of loss of residual renal function among new dialysis patients. J Am Soc Nephrol 2000;11: 556-564.

[50] Misra M, Vonesh E, Van Stone JC, Moore HL, Prowant B, Nolph KD. Effect of cause and time of dropout on the residual GFR: a comparative analysis of the decline of GFR on dialysis. Kidney Int 2001;59: 754-763.

[51] Jansen MAM, Hart AAM, Korevaar JC, Dekker FW, Boeschoten EW, Krediet RT. Predictors of the rate of decline of residual renal function in incident dialysis patients. Kidney Int 2002;62: 1046–1053.

[52] Fan S, Sayed RH, Davenport A. Extracellular volume expansion in peritoneal dialysis patients. Int J Artif Organs 2012;35(5): 338-345.

[53] Menon MK, Naimark DM, Bargman JM, Vas SI, Oreopoulos DG. Long-term blood pressure control in a cohort of peritoneal dialysis patients and its association with residual renal function. Nephrol Dial Transplant 2001;16: 2207-2213.

[54] Pérez-Flores I, Coronel F, Cigarrán S, Herrero JA, Calvo N. Relationship between residual renal function, inflammation, and anemia in peritoneal dialysis. Adv Perit Dial 2007;23: 140-143.

[55] Wang AY, Woo J, Wang M, Sea MM, Sanderson JE, Lui SF, Li PK. Important differentiation of factors that predict outcome in peritoneal dialysis with different degrees of residual renal function. Nephrol Dial Transplant 2005;20: 396-403.

[56] Ateş K, Nergizoğlu G, Keven K, Şen A, Kutlay S, Ertürk Ş, Duman N, Karatan O, Ertuğ AE. Effect of fluid and sodium removal on mortality in peritoneal dialysis patients. Kidney Int 2001; 60: 767-776.

[57] Konings CJ, Kooman JP, Schonck M, Struijk DG, Gladziwa U, Hoorntje SJ, van der Wall Bake AW, van der Sande FM, Leunissen KM. Fluid status in CAPD patients is related to peritoneal transport and residual renal function: evidence from a longitudinal study. Nephrol Dial Transplant 2003;18(4): 797-803.

[58] Khandelwal M, Kothari J, Krishnan M, Liakopoulos V, Tziviskou E, Sahu K, Chatalalsingh C, Bargman J, Oreopoulos D. Volume expansion and sodium balance in peritoneal dialysis patients. Part I: Recent concepts in pathogenesis. Adv Perit Dial 2003;19: 36–43.

[59] Enia G, Mallamaci F, Benedetto FA, Panuccio V, Parlongo S, Cutrupi S, Giacone G, Cottini E, Tripepi G, Malatino LS, Zoccali C. Long-term CAPD patients are volume expanded and display more severe left ventricular hypertrophy than haemodialysis patients. Nephrol Dial Transplant 2001;16: 1459–1464.

[60] Jokiniitty JM, Majahalme SK, Kähönen MA, Tuomisto MT, Turjanmaa VM. Pulse pressure is the best predictor of future left ventricular mass and change in left ventricular mass: 10 years of follow up. J Hypertens 2001;19: 2047-2054

[61] Levin A, Thompson CR, Ethier J, Carlisle EJ, Tobe S, Mendelssohn D, Burgess E, Jindal K, Barrett B, Singer J, Djurdjev O. Left ventricular mass index increase in early renal disease: impact of decline in hemoglobin. Am J Kidney Dis 1999;34(1): 125-134.

[62] Rigatto C, Foley RN, Kent GM, Guttmann R, Parfrey PS. Long-term changes in left ventricular hypertrophy after renal transplantation. Transplantation 2000;70(4): 570-575.

[63] Bammens B, Evenepoel P, Verbeke K, Vanrenterghem Y. Removal of middle molecules and protein-bound solutes by peritoneal dialysis and relation with uremic symptoms. Kidney Int 2003;64: 2238-2243.

[64] Pham NM, Recht NS, Hostetter TH, Meyer TW. Removal of the protein-bound solutes indican and p-cresol sulfate by peritoneal dialysis. Clin J Am Soc Nephrol 2008;3: 85-90.

[65] Amici G, Virga G, Da Rin G, Grandesso S, Vianello A, Gatti P, Bocci C. Serum beta-2 microglobulin level and residual renal function in peritoneal dialysis. Nephron 1993: 65: 469-471.

[66] Copley JB, Lindberg JS. Nontransplant therapy for dialysis-related amyloidosis. Semin Dial 2001;14: 94–98.

[67] Lopez-Menchero R, Miguel A, Garcia-Ramon R, Perez-Contreras J, Girbes V. Importance of residual renal function in continuous ambulatory peritoneal dialysis: its influence on different parameters of renal replacement treatment. Nephron 1999;83: 219-225.

[68] Erkan E, Moritz M, Kaskel F. Impact of residual renal function in children on hemodialysis. Pediatr Nephrol 2001;16: 858-861.

[69] Block GA, Hulbert-Shearon TE, Levin NW, Port FK. Association of serum phosphorus and calcium x phosphate product with mortality risk in chronic hemodialysis patients: a national study. Am J Kidney Dis 1998;31: 607-617.

[70] Wang AY, Woo J, Sea MM, Law MC, Lui SF, Li PK. Hyperphosphatemia in Chinese peritoneal dialysis patients with and without residual kidney function: what are the implications? Am J Kidney Dis 2004; 43: 712-720.

[71] Dervisoglu E, Altun EA, Kalender B, Caglayan C. Effects of Residual Renal Function on Clinical and Laboratory Features of Patients on Continuous Ambulatory Peritoneal Dialysis. BANTAO Journal 2007; 5(1): 36-39.

[72] Chung SH, Heimbürger O, Stenvinkel P, Qureshi AR, Lindholm B. Association between residual renal function, inflammation and patient survival in new peritoneal dialysis patients. Nephrol Dial Transplant 2003 Mar;18(3): 590-597.

[73] Wang AY, Lam CW, Wang M, Woo J, Chan IH, Lui SF, Sanderson JE, Li PK. Circulating soluble vascular cell adhesion molecule 1: relationships with residual renal function, cardiac hypertrophy, and outcome of peritoneal dialysis patients. Am J Kidney Dis 2005;45(4): 715-729.

[74] Pecoits-Filho R, Heimbürger O, Bárány P, Suliman M, Fehrman-Ekholm I, Lindholm B, Stenvinkel P. Associations between circulating inflammatory markers and residual renal function in CRF patients. Am J Kidney Dis 2003;41(6): 1212-1218.

[75] Shin SK, Noh H, Kang SW, Seo BJ, Lee IH, Song HY, Choi KH, Ha SK, Lee HY, Han DS. Risk factors influencing the decline of residual renal function in continuous ambulatory peritoneal dialysis patients. Perit Dial Int 1999;19(2): 138-142.

[76] Wang AY, Sea MM, Ip R, Law MC, Chow KM, Lui SF, Li PK, Woo J. Independent effects of residual renal function and dialysis adequacy on actual dietary protein, calorie, and other nutrient intake in patients on continuous ambulatory peritoneal dialysis. Am Soc Nephrol 2001;12(11): 2450-2457.

[77] Wang AY, Sea MM, Tang N, Sanderson JE, Lui SF, Li PK, Woo J. Resting energy expenditure and subsequent mortality risk in peritoneal dialysis patients. J Am Soc Nephrol 2004;15(12): 3134-3143.

[78] Scanziani R, Dozio B, Bonforte G, Surian M. Residual renal function and nutritional parameters in CAPD. Adv Perit Dial 1995;11: 106-109.

[79] Jones MR. Etiology of severe malnutrition: results of an international cross-sectional study in continuous ambulatory peritoneal dialysis patients. Am J Kidney Dis 1994;23: 412-420.

[80] Sipahioglu MH, Kucuk H, Unal A, Kaya MG, Oguz F, Tokgoz B, Oymak O, Utas C. Impact of arterial stiffness on adverse cardiovascular outcomes and mortality in peritoneal dialysis patients. Perit Dial Int 2012;32(1): 73-80.

[81] Wang AY, Wang M, Woo J, Lam CW, Lui SF, Li PK, Sanderson JE. Inflammation, residual kidney function, and cardiac hypertrophy are interrelated and combine adversely to enhance mortality and cardiovascular death risk of peritoneal dialysis patients. J Am Soc Nephrol 2004;15(8): 2186-2194.

[82] Szeto CC, Wong TY, Chow KM, Leung CB, Li PK. Are peritoneal dialysis patients with and without residual renal function equivalent for survival study? Insight from a retrospective review of the cause of death. Nephrol Dial Transplant 2003;18: 977-982.

[83] Bleyer A (author), Berns JS (section editor), Sheridan AM (deputy editor). Urine output and residual renal function in renal failure. http://www.uptodate.com/index/ (accessed 12 August 2012).

[84] Lameire N, Van Biesen W. The impact of residual renal function on the adequacy of peritoneal dialysis. Perit Dial Int 1997;17(2): 102-110.

[85] McKane W, Chandna SM, Tattersall JE, Greenwood RN, Farrington K. Identical decline of residual renal function in high-flux biocompatible hemodialysis and CAPD. Kidney Int 2002; 61: 256-265.

[86] Schiffl H, Lang SM, Fischer R. Ultrapure dialysis fluid slows loss of residual renal function in new dialysis patients. Nephrol Dial Transplant 2002;17: 1814–1818.

[87] McCarthy JT, Jenson BM, Squillace DP, Williams AW. Improved preservation of residual renal function in chronic hemodialysis patients using polysulfone dialyzers. Am J Kidney Dis 1997;29: 576-583.

[88] Hufnagel G, Michel C, Queffeulou G, Skhiri H, Damieri H, Mignon F. The influence of automated peritoneal dialysis on the decrease in residual renal function. Nephrol Dial Transplant 1999;14: 1224–1228.

[89] Michels WM, Verduijn M,Grootendorst DC, le Cessie S, Boeschoten EW, Dekker FW, Krediet RT; NECOSAD study group. Decline in residual renal function in automated compared with continuous ambulatory peritoneal dialysis. Clin J Am Soc Nephrol 2011;6(3): 537-542.

[90] Holley JL, Aslam N, Bernardini J, Fried L, Piraino B. The influence of demographic factors and modality on loss of residual renal function in incident peritoneal dialysis patients. Perit Dial Int 2001;21(3): 302-305.

[91] Cnossen TT, Usvyat L, Kotanko P, van der Sande FM, Kooman JP, Carter M, Leunissen KM, Levin NW. Comparison of outcomes on continuous ambulatory peritoneal dialysis versus automated peritoneal dialysis: results from a USA database. Perit Dial Int 2011;31(6): 679-684.

[92] Williams JD, Topley N, Craig KJ, Mackenzie RK, Pischetsrieder M, Lage C, Passlick-Deetjen J: The Euro-Balance Trial: the effect of a new biocompatible peritoneal dialysis fluid (balance) on the peritoneal membrane. Kidney Int 2004. 66; 408–418.

[93] Fan SL, Pile T, Punzalan S, Raftery MJ, Yaqoob MM. Randomized controlled study of biocompatible peritoneal dialysis solutions: effect on residual renal function. Kidney Int 2008;73: 200–206.

[94] Konings CJ, Kooman JP, Schonck M, Gladziwa U, Wirtz J, van den Wall Bake AW, Gerlag PG, Hoorntje SJ, Wolters J, van der Sande FM, Leunissen KM. Effect of icodextrin

on volume status, blood pressure and echocardiographic parameters: a randomized study. Kidney Int 2003;63: 1556–1563.

[95] Davies SJ, Woodrow G, Donovan K, Plum J, Williams P, Johansson AC, Bosselmann HP, Heimburger O, Simonsen O, Davenport A, Tranaeus A, Divino Filho JC. Icodextrin improves the fluid status of peritoneal dialysis patients: results of a double-blind randomized controlled trial. J Am Soc Nephrol 2003;14: 2338–2344.

[96] Davies SJ. Exploring new evidence of the clinical benefits of icodextrin solutions. Nephrol Dial Transplant 2006;21(2): 47–50.

[97] Medcalf JF, Harris KP, Walls J. Role of diuretics in the preservation of residual renal function in patients on continuous ambulatory peritoneal dialysis. Kidney Int 2001;59: 1128-1133.

[98] Li PK, Chow KM, Wong TY, Leung CB, Szeto CC. Effects of an angiotensin-converting enzyme inhibitor on residual renal function in patients receiving peritoneal dialysis. A randomized, controlled study. Ann Intern Med 2003;139: 105–112.

[99] Suzuki H, Kanno Y, Sugahara S, Okada H, Nakamoto H. Effects of an angiotensin II receptor blocker, valsartan, on residual renal function in patients on CAPD. Am J Kidney Dis 2004; 43: 1056-1064.

[100] Günal AI, Duman S, Ozkahya M, Töz H, Asçi G, Akçiçek F, Basçi A. Strict volume control normalizes hypertension in peritoneal dialysis patients. Am J Kidney Dis 2001;37: 588 –593.

[101] Baker RJ, Senior H, Clemenger M, Brown EA. Empirical aminoglycosides for peritonitis do not affect residual renal function. Am J Kidney Dis 2003;41(3): 670-675.

[102] Badve SV, Hawley CM, McDonald SP, Brown FG, Boudville NC, Wiggins KJ, Bannister KM, Johnson DW. Use of aminoglycosides for peritoneal dialysis-associated peritonitis does not affect residual renal function. Nephrol Dial Transplant 2012;27(1): 381-387.

[103] Moranne O, Willoteaux S, Pagniez D, Dequiedt P, Boulanger E. Effect of iodinated contrast agents on residual renal function in PD patients. Nephrol Dial Transplant 2006;21(4): 1040-1045.

[104] Dittrich E, Puttinger H, Schillinger M, Lang I, Stefenelli T, Hörl WH, Vychytil A. Effect of radio contrast media on residual renal function in peritoneal dialysis patients--a prospective study. Nephrol Dial Transplant 2006;21(5): 1334-1339.